FROM
STUDENT
TO
PHARMACIST:
Making the Transition

Notice

The author, editor, and publisher have made every effort to ensure the accuracy and completeness of the information presented in this book. However, the author, editor, and publisher cannot be held responsible for the continued currency of the information, any inadvertent errors or omissions, or the application of this information. Therefore, the author, editor, and publisher shall have no liability to any person or entity with regard to claims, loss, or damage caused or alleged to be caused, directly or indirectly, by the use of information contained herein.

L-22005-8-2012

FROM
STUDENT
TO
PHARMACIST:
Making the Transition

By Jennifer P. Askew

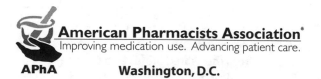

American Pharmacists Association®
Improving medication use. Advancing patient care.
APhA   **Washington, D.C.**

Managing and Content Editor: Vicki Meade, Meade Communications
Acquiring Editor: Sandra J. Cannon
Proofreader: Cathi Dunn MacRae
Editorial Assistant: Kellie Burton
Indexer: Jennifer Burton, Columbia Indexing Group
Cover Designer: Richard Muringer, APhA Creative Services
Layout and Graphics: Michele A. Danoff, Graphics by Design

© 2010 by the American Pharmacists Association
APhA was founded in 1852 as the American Pharmaceutical Association.

Published by the American Pharmacists Association
2215 Constitution Avenue, N.W.
Washington, DC 20037-2985
www.pharmacist.com

To comment on this book via email, send your message to the publisher at
aphabooks@aphanet.org.

Library of Congress Cataloging-in-Publication Data

Askew, Jennifer P.
  From student to pharmacist : making the transition / by Jennifer P.
Askew.
     p. ; cm.
  Includes bibliographical references and index.
  ISBN 978-1-58212-142-0
  1. Pharmacists—Vocational guidance. I. American Pharmacists Association. II. Title.
  [DNLM: 1. Career Choice. 2. Pharmacists. 3. Adaptation, Psychological.
QV 21 A835f 2010]
  RS122.5.A85 2010
  615'.1023—dc22
                              2010010062

How to Order This Book
Online: www.pharmacist.com/shop_apha
By phone: 800-878-0729 (from the United States and Canada)
VISA®, MasterCard®, and American Express® cards accepted

Contents

Preface

The idea for this book first came from the American Pharmacists Association (APhA) publications staff, who saw a poster I was presenting about the New Practitioners Network we'd recently established at the North Carolina Association of Pharmacists. As I talked with the APhA staff, I realized that student pharmacists and new practitioners really need a resource that addresses the changes and adjustments we go through when leaving pharmacy school.

When I was making that transition not so very long ago, I found myself wishing someone would give me the "nitty gritty" details. I had lots of wonderful resources, including books, pharmacy associations, mentors, coworkers, friends, and family to help me piece together the wisdom, knowledge, and assistance I needed. Even so, I felt I was largely in uncharted territory.

Some resources gave me great perspectives on one topic but had little to share on others. For example, one of my mentors—a relative, physician, and excellent businessman—coached me on negotiating job offers and other topics, but he's not a pharmacist and couldn't advise me from that standpoint. Another mentor, a fellow pharmacist, offered insights into the profession, but because he'd been in the same position for a long time, he had no recent experience with negotiating salary and benefits and couldn't really counsel me about it.

That's why I decided to put all my suggestions, ideas, and resources in one central place. My hope is that this book will make it easier for student pharmacists and new practitioners to find the guidance they need for success in the working world.

When I sat down to write, I realized that things had changed since I received my PharmD in 2003, and I'd lost some of that "student perspective." For example, my state no longer requires a hand-written board exam, and completing a PGY1 residency is now necessary before you can seek PGY2 specialty training. (I went straight from pharmacy school to a PGY2 program.)

An excellent student from Campbell University, Laurie Whalin, agreed to help me provide the student viewpoint, and she brainstormed with me about topics important to today's pharmacy school graduates. She wrote Chapters 2, 4, and 5 and provided material for other sections—and during the writing of this book, was making the transition from student to pharmacist herself. As the book goes to press, she's completing a PGY1 residency at my institution, New Hanover Regional Medical Center, as well as an MS degree in clinical research from Campbell University, where she earned her PharmD in 2009.

The topics covered in the book's 10 chapters follow the order in which you are likely to need them—such as preparing a CV or résumé (Chapter 4) before going out on job interviews (Chapter 5). I wrote in a conversational tone and, when relevant, inserted my personal experiences and suggestions, trying to make this book more fun to read than, say, your anatomy and physiology textbook. You can read the book straight through or use the table of contents and index to jump directly to the topics you need most. Keeping the book handy lets you quickly find advice and reference works relevant to whatever is going on at a certain stage, whether you're negotiating a salary or wondering how to improve your relationship with a coworker.

In this book I drew upon the wisdom of key experts, whose works are listed in the "further resources" boxes, and I blended in advice from the many people who have taught, guided, and inspired me. I hope you find this text a valuable addition to your professional bookshelf and can use it, not only during your transition from student to pharmacist, but well into your pharmacy career.

Let me know which portions are particularly helpful! And tell me if other topics or resources should be included in future editions.

Jennifer P. Askew
jennaskewunc@hotmail.com
March 2010

Acknowledgments

One of the best parts of writing this book is the opportunity to thank the people who helped make it possible. Some helped directly, some indirectly, and some simply put up with me during my first efforts as a book author.

To my husband, Russ, thank you for supporting me personally and professionally. I love that your glass is always more than half full and that you fill mine up when it gets a little low. I am so lucky to be married to my best friend.

To my parents—Paul, Nancy, Eddy, and Joy—thank you for all the love and support throughout the years. You were my first advisors and mentors, and my transition from child to adult, much less from student to pharmacist, would not have been as successful without you. And to my sister, Shawn, thank you for being such a great friend and confidante.

To my teachers, mentors, supervisors, and preceptors—especially my "ninja boss"—where would I be if you hadn't taken the time to impart all the lessons that form the foundation of this book? You made me into the health care professional I am today, and I'm not sure I'll ever be able to thank you enough.

To my friends, coworkers, employees, and colleagues, thank you for supporting me, believing in me, being patient with me, and helping me make it through the challenges I get myself into—like writing a book, for example.

And thank you to everyone who contributed quotes and "day in the life" stories (whose names are listed on the next page). You let me include your thoughts and experiences without reading the book first to assess its caliber—a true leap of faith. I hope you are happy with the result!

A special thanks goes to Laurie Whalin, whose input was a huge help. I'm very grateful.

Finally, I would like to thank the American Pharmacists Association for bringing this project to me and trusting me to take it on.

Contributors of quotes and stories:
Bruce Canaday
Stephen M. Feldman
Deborah A. Frieze
Amanda F. Fuller
Anna D. Garrett
Diane B. Ginsburg
Jean-Venable "Kelly" R. Goode
Erin Hendrick
Lucinda L. Maine
Anthony T. Pudlo
Jenna Reel
Megan Rose
John P. Rovers
Ryan Swanson
Laurie M. Whalin
Beth S. Williams
Abbie Crisp Williamson

Introduction: The Route Ahead

> "Build a network. When I was a new pharmacist, I wish someone had advised me to go out and meet doctors and nurses in the community—so you're not just a voice on the phone, but a professional they know and trust."
>
> —Jean-Venable "Kelly" R. Goode, professor and director, Community Pharmacy Practice and Residency Program, School of Pharmacy, Virginia Commonwealth University

When looking back on the five-plus years that have passed since I completed pharmacy school, I realize I was in no way prepared for my integration into the profession of pharmacy. My school, professors, preceptors, mentors, fellow students, and family all did their absolute best to make sure my transition was smooth, and I'm eternally grateful. But now that I'm a preceptor myself, I know that some things cannot be taught in a classroom or on a rotation.

I think I was most unprepared for the independence and personal accountability that come with the "real world" of practicing pharmacy. Let's face it; most of us accepted into pharmacy school were among the best of our undergraduate classes and tops in our high school coursework. We were expected to do well, get good grades, and make those who care about us proud. Evaluation and feedback were important parts of the learning process and there was a definitive end to each class, project, assignment, or school term.

In the first few years of my career, it felt strange that no one tested or evaluated me on a regular basis. Each month led to the next without clear-cut separation, and my boss conducted a performance review only once a year. I had to evaluate myself, ask for feedback when I needed it, and set my own goals and guidelines. I was now in charge of my career and where to go next. I hadn't understood how much everything in my world would change as I transitioned from student to pharmacist. I wish I'd sought more guidance about how to adapt and excel in my new surroundings.

Although it's unlikely that a book can truly get you ready to enter the profession, I hope the tips, advice, and resources on the coming pages will help ease your way through the first few years. Take a minute to read the questions that Laurie Whalin, a student pharmacist, poses in Box 1-1. Have you wondered the same things? This book should answer many of your questions.

Knowing It All

I chose the profession of pharmacy because it's so diverse, giving me the ability to work in research, patient care, management, or academia. Yet pharmacy's wonderful variety also makes it difficult to prepare student pharmacists for what awaits on the other side of graduation. Your future might involve taking care of patients—at a pharmacy counter or by the bedside—or it might look more like a desk job, for example. Your school gave you an excellent foundation for these roles, but each option requires different skill sets. There is no way you will know everything you need by the time you receive your diploma.

You've been introduced to the key information and skills, but you haven't mastered them all. This is normal—and you'll cope by filling gaps in your knowledge base when they arise. Sometimes the remedy might be as simple as looking up the answer to a drug-related question in *Goodman and Gilman's* or as complex as seeking additional training. Gaps in your knowledge base do not make you an inadequate health care professional—they make you human—and it's important to recognize that sometimes you won't have all the information you need.

Does this mean you can give yourself permission to remain static rather than staying on top of new information and skills? Absolutely not. Continuous professional development is an integral part of being a pharmacist. It's your responsibility to supplement and expand your knowledge throughout your career.

Where to Focus?

Students ask, "Are there certain subjects I should focus on more than others?" The answer really depends on how much you know about what awaits you on the other side of graduation. For example, if you already plan to work in your family's pharmacy business and eventually take it over, you can certainly concentrate on subjects that will better prepare you for that task. If you've known for a long time that you want to work "at the bench top" doing research, you might need different courses and experience to get ready. Advisors, mentors, and preceptors within your school or community can help you tailor your elective coursework and rotations to your needs.

You may be thinking, "But what about those of us who don't know what we want to do?" Well, that's probably the perspective I know best—because I had no idea, other than that I wanted to use my knowledge of medicine to make a difference in my community. Many different career paths could fit that description.

I chose pharmacy because I want to work in health care, because nursing and medicine didn't seem right for me, and because I preferred having many different options for specialization. I decided to try on as many hats as I could during my time as a student pharmacist to see which one fit the best.

It's okay for you to tell friends, family, professors, preceptors, and colleagues that you just aren't sure yet which career "hat" is the right fit—as long as you're still trying them on. As discussed further in Chapter 3, don't choose what you think is pleasing to your mentors. Your path in pharmacy is up to you. You have many ways to get a taste of various roles before you make a long-term commitment.

Tools to Build, Skills to Develop

As you transition into the world of professional pharmacy, some things are applicable to everyone, regardless of your career path—such as developing your interviewing skills, deciding whether to seek advanced training and choosing the right program for you, and building an effective résumé, curriculum vitae, and portfolio. Chapters 4 and 5 provide advice on these matters and refer you to helpful resources.

I remember that, for me, one of the hardest things about creating my résumé was looking objectively at my achievements and figuring out how to highlight them. I felt as if I hadn't proven myself yet—but actually, by the time we graduate, we've already had successes we can tout, such as projects we've initiated, presentations we've given, and contributions we've made during internships and rotations. We have to sort through our long list of activities and pull out the ones that speak loudest about our strengths so we can sell ourselves effectively.

I'm sure you know you need a résumé or CV, but you probably haven't thought about many other areas this book covers, such how to develop your leadership and communication skills, strategies for adjusting to the workplace, and ways to cope with being the new kid on the block. The latter chapters in the book cover these topics.

When I was a student, I didn't realize the huge role that communication skills play in the workplace. Being able to interact successfully, get your message across, and listen to others is crucial to career success, no matter whether you spend more time with patients or with other health care professionals. Trust me—even if your written and oral communication skills are above average, there are aspects of interpersonal communication you can and must continue to develop.

I'll never forget the first time I had to give a major presentation to hospital administrators. On the surface, this task may seem easy if you've given presentations in school before. It was different, though, because my audience was not pharmacists, professors, or students—it was executives. These very intelligent people had a limited knowledge of pharmacy practice. I had to figure out how to offer enough information to get my point across without inundating them—and without giving the impression that I thought my audience wasn't smart. I'd never had to adjust details and delivery in this way before. The stakes were very high. The presentation was worth much more than a grade in a class; it determined whether I could begin a big project that was really important to me.

Leadership skills are crucial in health care, whether you choose a management position or not. At some point in your new career, in some capacity, you'll find yourself directing or guiding others. And you'll draw on leadership skills daily even if you simply work alongside pharmacy technicians and other support staff.

Adjusting to your new schedule is another key learning task. Once you enter practice, you'll find it's very different from what you've experienced so far, even during rotations. You may consider yourself a pro at balancing the personal and professional aspects of student life; even so, sometimes you'll struggle to fit everything in when you're in the workplace full time. It's something I grapple with constantly as a practitioner, preceptor, manager, committee member, and even as a daughter, sister, friend, and wife.

You'll no longer have the immediate support of professors, preceptors, and classmates that you've been accustomed to. You'll have advisors, mentors, and colleagues to turn to for professional and personal advice, but first you'll need to build a network of resources. If you don't think about this issue ahead of time, support may not be there when you need it.

There isn't one "right" way to assimilate into your new work environment or ensure your success in pharmacy. But there are many things you must do to move ahead in a positive way. The transformation from student to professional pharmacist is rarely smooth or easy. You'll encounter bumps along the route, your expectations will change, and many times you'll have to look deep inside yourself. It's all part of the growing process. The pointers in this book, the people in your network, and the knowledge and skills you established in pharmacy school will help launch you toward your life as a productive and respected pharmacist.

School vs. the Real World – The Student Perspective
by Laurie M. Whalin

As we sit in class, study for exams, prepare projects, and participate in student professional organizations, it can be hard to think of the day when we'll no longer be consumed with student life. But the time when we will be practicing pharmacists is much closer than we think.

As I write this, I'm in my last year of pharmacy school completing my final experiential rotations. For a long time, the idea of being an *actual* pharmacist seemed as far from reality as winning the lottery. But now that graduation is near, I keep wondering, "How do I make the transition from school to the real world? How do I change from student to new practitioner?"

I have so many questions. How much information that I study for each exam will I use in practice each day? I'm fixated on the details so I perform well on exams, but I don't know if that's appropriate or even feasible for a busy pharmacist. With so many drugs, interactions, and side effects to be aware of, is it important to memorize details? Or should I acquire a baseline working knowledge—and then know where to look for more information?

During school we're inundated with an overwhelming amount of material. We find ourselves cramming, only to forget the information as we move on to the next subject, concept, or exam. What does this mean for our future? Will we be adequately prepared?

In discussions with my classmates, many concerns come up. How can you tailor your learning to one setting when the pharmacy profession has so many options to choose from? If you know you want to practice in a community pharmacy, should you focus more on some subjects than others? The information we are learning is crucial to our careers and the welfare of our future patients—but what is the best way to reinforce these vital concepts? Will we ever really be able to apply the knowledge we gained during pharmacy school in a real-life practice setting?

While dwelling in the pharmacy school "bubble," we're told what to learn, by when, and how. Yet the minute we receive our diplomas and step into the world, no one will be holding our hands. It will be up to us to figure out how to stay abreast of everything. With new drug approvals and fresh information from clinical trials coming in almost daily, how will we stay up to date while handling all the responsibilities of a practicing

continued on page 6

Box 1-1

continued

pharmacist? And once we've sorted through the information, how do we apply it to our practice and our patients?

The professors, researchers, clinical specialists, and other experts who surround us while we're in pharmacy school typically have an "open door" policy, allowing pharmacy students to stop in anytime we need advice. After graduation, when that door closes, who can we turn to when we have questions? Having developed my basic pharmacy skills in a supportive environment, I wonder how to handle having less personal support. I'll be transitioning to a situation that isn't student-centered, in which my needs and growth are no longer the focus. The organization and the patients will be the priority.

What about the concept of "professionalism"? Is it the same in the working world as it is in school? And how do we change our routines from finishing class in the early afternoon and cramming at night, changing classes every hour and switching courses every six months, to a structured workplace—40 hours a week in the same location with the same people? How do we keep our day-to-day professional activities interesting? How do we handle our shortcomings, mistakes, and failures—which are bound to happen?

In pharmacy school, poor performance on an exam or project only affects ourselves, but in a practice setting, mistakes can have consequences for colleagues or patients. In school, we might choose to sacrifice an A on a quiz to go out with friends one night, but in our careers, A-level work will be required all the time. How do we learn to have fun without compromising our success? How do we balance personal and professional priorities?

I still don't know many of the answers, even though I'll graduate soon. This book should help new practitioners like me—and you—transition from school to the real world.

—Laurie M. Whalin earned her PharmD in 2009 from Campbell University School of Pharmacy.

Board Licensure

Laurie M. Whalin
2009 PharmD Recipient
Campbell University School of Pharmacy

So, we've come all this way. We've endured long nights of studying, passed intense pharmacotherapy exams, and completed our experiential rotations. Now one big thing stands between us and the pharmacy career we've always wanted: the NAPLEX.

The North American Pharmacist Licensure Exam (NAPLEX) was developed by the National Association of Boards of Pharmacy (NABP) to help boards of pharmacy assess whether a pharmacy school graduate has the minimum competence and knowledge to practice pharmacy. It is an essential step in becoming licensed to practice pharmacy in your state.

As a 2009 pharmacy graduate who took the NAPLEX just after graduating, I remember all too clearly the feelings of anxiety and pressure, which grew as the exam date arrived. Understanding the test format, knowing about helpful resources, and following the advice of others who previously took the exam helped me feel more confident, and I'm sure will help you, too.

This chapter provides background and tips regarding the NAPLEX and the Multistate Pharmacy Jurisprudence Examination (MPJE), required steps on the road to being a pharmacy practitioner in most states. And Box 2-4 at the end of the chapter talks a little about managing the stress you're sure to feel as you study, sit for, and await the results of these tests.

"Licensure exams are just one piece of the assessment process. Once you pass, the training wheels come off—and you must maintain competency throughout your pharmacy career. You're not just studying for a test, you're preparing for practice and for continual professional development."

—Diane B. Ginsburg, clinical professor and assistant dean for student affairs, College of Pharmacy, University of Texas at Austin; editor-in-chief, ASHP's PharmPrep: Interactive Case-Based Board Review

The NAPLEX

The NAPLEX is a multiple-choice examination of 185 questions, which is delivered in a computer-adaptive format. In simple terms, this means that the computer selectively chooses the next question based on how you performed on previous questions. If you answer a question correctly, a more difficult question follows. If you answer incorrectly, an easier question follows.

Because computer-adaptive tests are tailored to the examinee based on how he or she answers previous questions, they allow for a shorter examination. Of the 185 questions, 150 count toward your score. The other 35 are pilot questions that are being evaluated for their inclusion on future exams. These questions are distributed throughout the test so you will not be able to distinguish them from scored questions.

Competency Areas

The NAPLEX is divided into three areas, defined by "competency statements." Competency statements articulate the skills and knowledge you are supposed to have acquired before sitting for the exam and before becoming a pharmacist. The competency statements ultimately provide a breakdown of what is covered on the examination. Although the test questions are not separated into competency areas on the examination, having a solid understanding of the competencies gives you a much greater chance of success on the exam.

Area 1: Assure Safe and Effective Pharmacotherapy and Optimize Therapeutic Outcomes

This area, covering approximately 54% of the exam, tests your ability to:
- Evaluate disease state presentations.
- Identify patient-specific information that may affect treatment.
- Evaluate the appropriateness of pharmacologic therapy including dose and dosage forms.
- Monitor for safety and efficacy.
- Provide patient education.

Area 2: Assure Safe and Accurate Preparation and Dispensing of Medication

This area, covering approximately 35% of the exam, tests your ability to:
- Perform calculations necessary to compound or administer medications.
- Identify drugs by brand or generic name.
- Determine if medications are commercially available and whether they can be obtained without a prescription.
- Determine equivalence between manufactured products and describe packaging, storage, and handling of medications.

Area 3: Provide Health Care Information and Promote Public Health
Covering the remaining 11% of the exam, this area tests your ability to:
- Apply information to promote health care.
- Evaluate the reliability of information from references.
- Evaluate the sufficiency of experimental design.
- Apply statistical tests.
- Recommend products for self-care.

When the exam was updated in 2005, a new section was added that includes dietary supplements, with a focus on adverse reactions and toxicities.

Format

A substantial number of questions on the NAPLEX appear in a case-based format. This means you are presented with a patient "profile" that includes such information as the patient's history, medications, and allergies. You are then asked a series of questions, and you must refer to the profile to be able to answer them correctly.

The remaining questions stand alone. In other words, you should be able to obtain all the necessary information from the question itself in order to select the correct answer.

Throughout the test, keep in mind that there may be more than one correct answer—what you need to do is choose the *best* answer. The test employs both questions with single answers and multi-response questions, where looking for the best combination is critical.

How to Prepare

Key questions I hear tossed around when classmates discuss board preparation are, "When should I start studying?" and "How should I prepare?" Answers vary, but the common theme is don't wait until the last minute.

Pharmsuccess.com, a website that markets practice tests, recommends preparing for at least two months before taking the NAPLEX, and studying for about four hours per day. James C. Eoff III, a co-editor of *The APhA Complete Review for Pharmacy*, recommends in his introduction that you begin a serious review no less than four to six weeks before your exam date. Anecdotal responses from recently licensed pharmacists with whom I talked suggest that you should spend anywhere from 30 days to four months preparing.

Many resources exist to help you prepare to take the NAPLEX. Some of the most popular choices are outlined in Box 2-1.

Box 2-1

Selected Resources for NAPLEX Preparation

The APhA Complete Review for Pharmacy

(Gourley DR, Eoff JC, eds. 7th ed. Washington, DC: American Pharmacists Association; 2010.)
Primarily, this review text summarizes therapeutic principles, including disease states
and treatments, as well as basic pharmaceutical principles such as calculations,
dosage forms, compounding, and kinetics.
- Uses an abbreviated outline format to help you recall information easily.
- Includes lists of key points at the end of each chapter, along with answers and
  explanations.
- Has summary tables of the major drug categories.
- Reviews the brand/generic names of the top 200 drugs.
- Provides drug charts with dosage schedules and dosage forms.
- Is accompanied by a CD-ROM with almost 1000 questions and detailed answers.

Appleton and Lange Review of Pharmacy

(Hall GD, Reiss BS. 9th ed. New York: McGraw-Hill Companies, Inc.; 2007.)
This resource consists mainly of sample test questions and answers, allowing the user
to practice using the format of the actual examination itself.
- Contains patient medication profiles in addition to more than 1000 questions similar
  to those on the NAPLEX.
- CD-ROM is available for an additional cost, containing comprehensive, simulated
  practice exams to help you pinpoint your strengths and weaknesses. This CD-ROM
  simulates the test, allows for the creation of customized tests, and provides areas for
  saving notes for later study.

ASHP's PharmPrep Online

(www.pharmpreponline.com)
This interactive, case-based, online program covers most of the disease states you are
likely to encounter on the NAPLEX.
- You utilize real-life situations to practice your skills for providing drug information to
  patients and providers, performing calculations, dispensing, and compounding.
- Includes strategies for successful test taking, plus thorough explanations of both
  correct and incorrect answers.

continued on page 11

Box 2-1

continued

Comprehensive Pharmacy Review

(Shargel L, Mutnick AH, Souney PF, et al. 7th ed. Philadelphia: Lippincott Williams & Wilkins; 2009.)

In this book, chapters written by more than 50 specialists cover all subjects in the pharmacy curriculum, including pharmacology, pharmaceutics, and pharmacy practice.

- Includes sections on Federal law and drug-drug/drug-nutrient interactions.
- Provides exam tips and strategies.
- Printed paperback, CD-ROM version, and practice exams are available for purchase separately or as a bundled package.

Employer Board Reviews

Many future employers, such as large chain pharmacies, offer free board review sessions for interns who have signed early contracts. If you have committed early to a company, check with your human resources department or district manager to see if the company offers such programs to recent graduates.

Kaplan Test Prep and Admissions

(www.kaptest.com)

Kaplan, an educational publishing and online learning company, offers several resources to help you prepare for the NAPLEX:

The Kaplan NAPLEX Review: The Complete Guide to Licensing Exam Certification for Pharmacists—a comprehensive review of all the medications covered on the exam.

- Contains easy-to-use reference tables.
- Includes Kaplan's proven study tips.
- Features an efficient time-management tool including an estimated time for review for each subject.

Kaplan's NAPLEX Qbank and Lecture Notes—a combination print and online source of content and practice questions.

- Offers more than 400 pages of exam review content.
- Includes practical lessons on test-taking skills and strategies.
- Three months of access to a continuously updated question bank of more than 1000 exam questions can be customized by discipline.
- Onscreen feedback graphically displays your performance.
- Gives detailed explanations about why the right answer is correct and the distracters are incorrect.

continued on page 12

Box 2-1

continued

NAPLEX Review Course—an intensive, three-day, live lecture-style program that covers all NAPLEX competencies, relevant curriculum, and sample questions.
— Reviews medical terminology and drug references.
— Features exam-relevant drug interaction guide and calculation review.
— Contains complete set of lecture notes and review exercises to practice at home.

Pharmacy School Board Reviews

Schools of pharmacy often hold board review sessions for graduating students before the graduation date arrives. If your school does not offer such a program, contact surrounding schools, which regularly let outside students participate in review sessions for a nominal fee.

Pre-NAPLEX

(www.prenaplex.com)
NABP offers this 50-question online practice test to help students familiarize themselves with taking the NAPLEX. It contains questions used on previous exams, so this may be one of the best ways to estimate how you will perform on the actual NAPLEX. The Pre-NAPLEX is not intended as a study guide, but instead should be used to familiarize yourself with the look and feel of the test and the formatting of questions.
— Costs $50 per test; you are only permitted to take a total of two tests.
— You have 70 minutes to complete the 50 questions.
— As with the NAPLEX, you are not allowed to go back to a question once you have submitted an answer.
— Complete the entire exam to receive a score report, which you may keep for your records.

The Day of the Exam

You've been studying for weeks. You've gone through hundreds of example questions and even taken several practice exams. You've registered for the exam and now test day is here. So what should you expect?

First, you should have received a scheduled test time from Pearson, which runs the testing centers where the NAPLEX is administered. Plan to arrive at least 30 minutes prior to this scheduled time, which will allow sufficient time for registration and administration details.

It's important to remember that if you are more than 30 minutes *late* to your testing appointment, the testing center can cancel your registration, keep your fee, and require you to reapply to take the exam. So be on time!

If for some reason the testing center is running behind and you have to wait more than 30 minutes to take the exam, you can choose to continue waiting or to reschedule for another day at no additional charge.

You must bring two forms of identification with you to the testing center:
–   A picture ID containing your signature (driver's license, passport).
–   An ID that contains at least your signature (credit cards, military ID).

After your identification has been verified, your photograph and fingerprint will be taken. The testing site administrator will then give you a locker where you can keep your belongings during the exam, as nothing is allowed in the testing center with you. The administrator will also tell you where to keep your ID because it must be verified each time you leave or re-enter the testing room.

Once you enter the testing room and are taken to your work station, you will not be permitted to leave the room unless the testing administrator gives you permission. If you need to leave the room for any reason, the time you are absent will be deducted from the total testing time of four hours and 15 minutes. So use your time wisely. You get a scheduled 10-minute break after two hours of testing; keep this in mind to help you plan any additional breaks you may choose to take.

The testing administrator will provide you with the following:
–   Erasable note board
–   Dry-erase pen
–   Five-function on-screen calculator

Most testing centers resemble computer skills labs; you are probably familiar with these already. There will be desks, or cubicles, with a typical PC computer for each scheduled applicant. Make sure you are comfortable with the computer screen, keyboard, and mouse before beginning the exam, as you will not want to waste any test-taking time requesting assistance.

The questions will be presented on the computer screen in front of you. There is no way to skip questions and return to them. You have to answer each question in the order in which it is presented.

Also, if you prefer a hand-held calculator, be sure to ask the test administrator; these should be available at most testing centers and can be requested at any time.

Pace yourself throughout the testing period. With 185 questions to answer in four hours, the average amount of time available for each question is 1.5 minutes. Don't get bogged down on any one question. Box 2-2 gives a quick summary of tips for NAPLEX day.

Prepare wisely, and you should have no problems. Remember, you've been getting ready for this test for almost four years now. Take a deep breath and relax.

Box 2-2

Quick Tips for NAPLEX Day

— Arrive at the testing site at least 30 minutes early.
— If you arrive more than 30 minutes late, the testing center can cancel your registration.
— Bring two forms of identification: a picture ID with your signature (e.g., driver's license or passport) and another ID with your signature (e.g., credit cards or military ID).
— Be prepared to have your photograph and fingerprint taken.
— Put your belongings in the supplied locker. (Nothing is allowed in the testing center during the exam.)
— The test administrator will tell you where to keep your ID, which must be verified each time you leave or re-enter the testing room.
— You will be given a noteboard, pen, and five-function on-screen calculator—or hand-held version if you ask for one.
— Pace yourself. Total testing time is four hours and 15 minutes, with a scheduled 10-minute break after two hours of testing. That's 1.5 minutes per question.
— Because you will be penalized for any questions you leave unanswered, answer every question, even if you must make an educated guess.
— Remember, you've been getting ready for four years. Take a deep breath, relax, and get started.

NAPLEX Scoring

To pass the NAPLEX, you must achieve a score of 75 or greater. Your reported score is not a percentage of the questions you answered correctly. It is a calculated score based on your ability level during the exam, which is compared to the minimum acceptable ability level established for the exam. In other words, the score you receive is an independent value based on an algorithm that considers:
— The number of questions you answered correctly.
— The level of difficulty of the questions you answered correctly.

To receive a score on the NAPLEX, you must answer at least 162 of the exam's 185 questions. Unlike other standardized tests you may have taken in the past, you are penalized for questions you leave unanswered, so make sure you answer every question, even if you must make an educated guess.

Scores are reported from the NABP to the respective boards of pharmacy on a daily basis, and from there, scores are usually reported to students within two business days. Some boards of pharmacy will allow you to access the scores online; some will allow you to pick up your scores from the office; others will provide your results over the phone; and some will mail the scores to your home. The best way to determine how you will be notified of your test results is to check with the boards of pharmacy in the states for which you are seeking licensure. This information is often available on board of pharmacy websites.

If you do not pass the exam, you receive a detailed diagnostic report that examines your performance in each of the major areas. Those who do not pass can retake the NAPLEX 91 days after the date they took the previous exam.

The Multi-State Pharmacy Jurisprudence Examination (MPJE)

Like the NAPLEX, the MPJE is a computer-adaptive examination; as you take the test it selectively chooses your questions based on your responses to the previous questions. Developed by the NABP in conjunction with state boards of pharmacy, the MPJE combines federal and state-specific law questions to serve as the state law exam.

Most but not all states require the MPJE. You can take the MPJE and NAPLEX in any order you wish depending on test site availability. I recommend allowing yourself some time between tests so you can focus on preparing for each test individually. However, if it works for you and time allows, you can take both tests in the same day.

The MPJE consists of 90 multiple-choice questions, of which 75 count toward your score and 15 are pilot questions being tested for future exams. Box 2-3 lists some resources to help you prepare.

Competency Areas

The MPJE is divided into three main areas that correspond with competency statements defining the skills and knowledge you are expected to have. As with the NAPLEX, these areas will not be separated into areas on the exam itself; you will simply answer questions as they appear in front of you on the computer screen.

Area 1: Pharmacy Practice
Encompassing nearly 78% of the entire exam, the Pharmacy Practice section assesses your ability to identify the following:

— Legal responsibilities of the pharmacist and pharmacy personnel.
— Legal requirements of prescriptions and drug orders.
— Necessary procedures surrounding drug distribution, dispensing, and record keeping.
This portion of the exam has a heavy focus on controlled substances.

Area 2: Licensure, Registration, Certification, and Operational Requirements
Approximately 17% of the questions on the exam will relate to area 2. This portion:
— Assesses your knowledge of the necessary qualifications, examinations, and requirements of all personnel involved in manufacturing, distributing, or dispensing prescription and nonprescription medications.
— Contains questions regarding registration and operational requirements of various practice settings.

Area 3: Regulatory Structure and Terms
Covering the remaining 5% of the exam, these questions focus on:
— Defining terms found within the laws and rules governing pharmacy.
— The responsibilities of various agencies that enforce laws and rules governing pharmacy.

Box 2-3

Selected Resources for MPJE Preparation

Employer Law Reviews
Many future employers, such as large chain pharmacies, offer free law review sessions for interns who have signed early contracts. If you have committed to a company for employment, check with your human resources department or district manager to see if the company offers such programs to recent graduates.

Expert Law Reviews
Many states have pharmacy law experts who will hold review sessions for graduating students preparing to take the MPJE. These reviews are normally intense, full-day sessions lasting one to two days, often held at surrounding schools of pharmacy. It is best to schedule your MPJE within one to two weeks of this type of review, because students typically report better scores when their expert law review was very recent.

Guide to Federal Pharmacy Law
(Hall GD, Reiss BS. 6th ed. Boynton Beach, Fla: Apothecary Press; 2009.)
This pharmacy law review is a comprehensive study guide containing the newest federal statutes and regulations.

continued on page 17

Box 2-3

continued

– Includes updates on Medicare Part D, controlled substance ordering systems (CSOS), medication therapy management (MTM), and Health Insurance Portability and Accountability Act (HIPAA) regulations.
– Contains over 350 practice questions with detailed answers.

Pharmacy and Federal Drug Law Review: A Patient Profile Approach
(Kosegarten D, Pisano D. New York: McGraw-Hill Companies, Inc.; 2006.)
This review book is designed to help students prepare for both the NAPLEX and the MPJE.
– Offers more than 250 real-life case study reviews of disease states, pharmaco-therapeutics, pharmaceutics, pharmacology, and other basic science refreshers.
– Provides an overview of federal pharmacy law.
– Contains over 2000 practice questions with answers and explanations, including tips on how to answer the "tricky" questions.

Pharmacy Law: Textbook and Review
(Feinberg D. 1st ed. New York: McGraw-Hill Companies, Inc.; 2008.)
An accessible, concise review of pharmacy law that is ideal for both coursework and MPJE preparation.
– Covers relevant laws, rules, and regulations.
– Highlights the distinctions between state and federal law, where appropriate.
– Contains a comprehensive set of more than 450 practice questions formatted in the style of the MPJE, along with answers.
– Comes with a supplementary CD-ROM that contains a "board-simulating" interface, allowing the user to answer sample test questions in the format of the actual examination.

Pharmacy Practice and the Law
(Abood RR. 5th ed. Sudbury, Mass: Jones and Bartlett Publishers; 2008.)
A useful resource for teaching the facts and stimulating critical thinking in pharmacy law, the latest version of this best-selling text includes updated material in every chapter.
– The latest on HIPAA, Medicare Part D, and other new regulations.
– Comprehensive glossary.
– Additional review questions and "practice scenarios."

Pharmacy School Law Reviews
Schools of pharmacy often hold law review sessions before graduation for graduating students. If your school does not offer such a program, contact surrounding schools, which regularly let outside students participate in review sessions for a nominal fee.

Scoring

To pass the MPJE you must achieve a score of 75 or greater. As with the NAPLEX, this score is not a percentage of the questions you answered correctly, but is an independent value that is calculated based on the number of questions you answered correctly and the difficulty of those questions.

You must answer at least 77 of the 90 questions on the exam to receive a score. If you don't answer all 90 questions, a penalty is applied to your score, so it's crucial that you attempt to provide an answer for every question.

Box 2-4

Manage Your Stress
by Jennifer P. Askew

Now that you have some tools and tips to prepare for your licensure examinations, I'll share the good news—most schools of pharmacy report pass rates of over 90% for both the MPJE and the NAPLEX. Those are great odds! (If you want to see the statistics for yourself, check out NABP's website at www.nabp.net. Look under Licensure Examinations for the link called "School Pass Rates Statistical Analysis.")

I recommend that you *do not* study most of the day before the exam. Cramming on the last day or spending long hours reviewing the information can backfire because it intensifies your anxiety level. When you study over many weeks or months you place the information in your long-term memory, which is more permanent, whereas cramming puts it in short-term memory, which tends to fail under stress. If you've been studying several hours per day in advance of the exam, you know the material. The day before the test, find ways to relax. Go out for a nice early dinner. Get some exercise. Hit the sack at a reasonable hour for a good night's sleep.

Once the test is over, stay busy in the days that follow while you wait for your score. Many pharmacists find those days more stressful than the days spent preparing for the exams. Pick up a shift at work or treat yourself to social time with friends or family. Worrying about how you performed will not change the result. If you "did your homework" and prepared as much as you were able, you did your best.

Although it may seem like the end of the world if you fail one or both examinations, it isn't. You can retake the NAPLEX after 91 days and the MPJE after 30 days.

continued on page 19

Box 2-4

continued

Some states also require that you take their own board examination before you're granted your license to practice pharmacy in that state. A few years ago, when I took my exams, I honestly found my written state exam much more stressful than the computer-administered NAPLEX and MPJE. It was given to all applicants in one huge room with the members of the board of pharmacy sitting facing us, as supervisors.

Seating was alphabetical. I was stationed front and center, with the board observing from a platform directly in front of my table. This test contained short-answer questions and required checking simulated prescriptions for potential errors. The exam required hand-grading, so the waiting period to receive our scores was much longer than for the NAPLEX or MPJE. And if we didn't pass, the test was not offered again for about six months.

I'll be honest. When I got to my car after that exam was over, I had a good cry. I couldn't even begin to guess how well I'd done. I figured I'd botched it, and most of my classmates felt the same way. But in the end, my scores were very high. So remember, even if you come out of an exam feeling stressed and disappointed, try to be optimistic. You probably did better than you think.

Testing has come a long way in the few years since I took my licensure exams. Many tests are offered in more locations; they are tailored to the individual examinee; and results are available faster. As long as you take the time to understand the exams and prepare for them properly, you are likely to pass with flying colors.

Choosing a Career Path

"Finding your career is like sailing. Let the wind carry you and end up someplace. Or choose a destination, plot your course, set the sails—and be ready to change direction based on tides or weather. Planning and flexibility will get you where you want to go."

—Bruce Canaday, clinical professor, Pharmacy Practice and Experiential Education, University of North Carolina Eshelman School of Pharmacy; director, Department of Pharmacotherapy, SEAHEC

One of the best things about the profession of pharmacy is that so many career options await you. With all the paths to choose from, you're sure to find one that's right for you. The best advice I can give to a student pharmacist is to determine *your* priorities and *your* best fit.

That may seem like common sense, but it's easy to be swayed by the opinions of others, particularly those you see as mentors, supporters, and role models. Seriously. Have you decided you want to go into clinical pharmacy? How about retail? Or are you sure you want to be in research? Now, think about *why* you want to pursue this path. Is it because someone you admire has a successful career in that field? Or someone important to you advised you that this path would be a good fit for you?

The only good reason to choose a certain direction is because you truly feel it's the right one for you—something you will enjoy.

I struggled with confusion over which path to follow while I was a student pharmacist—experiencing feelings similar to Laurie Whalin's (see Box 3-1). In fact, even though I graduated from pharmacy school seven years ago, at times I still don't know what I want to be when I "grow up."

For a long time, I wanted a career in the pharmaceutical industry because a best friend from my undergraduate studies, who was a year ahead of me in pharmacy school, told me I was suited for this type of work. Although work in the industry is an excellent option, after completing an internship in this area I decided it wasn't the best fit for *me*.

Thoroughly exploring your personal answer to the question, "What work environment is best for me?" is as important as studying for that upcoming biochemistry test. And if you're anything like me, this is the hardest type of homework. It's not a project you can finish in one sitting. There is no format, deadline, or due date. You don't even have to do it at all, if you choose not to.

In fact, trying to answer the question about the best work environment reminds me of the reflection statements we had to do in pharmaceutics lab about "touchy-feely" topics, such as how does it feel to counsel a patient? Or what was it like to present a drug monograph? I always rushed through those assignments at the last minute just to put something on paper, more interested in learning hard science and getting the asthma guidelines down before the next therapeutics exam. But now I know that to get the most out of your pharmacy career, you must make the effort to really understand who you are and where you will thrive.

Box 3-1

What Kind of Pharmacist Am I? The Student Perspective
by Laurie M. Whalin

One reason I decided on pharmacy as a profession is the number of diverse practice settings available. But as I write this, I'm on the verge of graduating and I have so many prospects before me, I can't help but think, how could I possibly choose just one?

Some students know, before even entering pharmacy school, exactly where they want to practice and what type of pharmacist they want to be. Where does that leave the rest of us?

Throughout my experiential rotations this past year, I kept waiting for a light to turn on in my head saying, "This is it! This is the type of pharmacist I should be." But as the months went on I felt more confused. Each time I was exposed to a new area—hospital practice, ambulatory care, long-term care, and then the specialties, including internal medicine, cardiology, and infectious disease—I really liked each one.

So if you are feeling this same way, trust me, you are not alone. You may find yourself wondering how you can narrow the choices to find the career that's right for you. Is there homework you should complete to begin the process of determining a career path? Should you seek residency training or directly enter the work force? Even though it can sometimes feel like homework, I have already begun to use formalized assessments and other tools, such as those described in this chapter, to identify the next steps that are right for me.

Write 'Likes' and 'Dislikes' to Get Started

I've found that writing down my thoughts makes reflecting feel more concrete and useful. When I'm finished, I have a product. And later I can go back and edit it when I discover something new to add. Maybe some people can make major life assessments all in their heads, without ever putting pen to paper. But chances are, writing your thoughts will benefit you, just as it does me.

Even if you're stymied by the belief that you don't yet have enough experience to narrow your career options, the truth is, you have more than you think.

Sit down with a notepad and a cup of coffee. Make a list of "likes" and "dislikes" about your past work, school, and life experiences. For example:
– Do you like to work in groups or would you rather work alone?
– Do you want each day to be similar or do you prefer a new and completely different challenge each day?
– Do you enjoy brief, frequent interactions with lots of people or do you prefer extended interactions with just a few people?
– Would you like to work one-on-one with patients or would working in a more "behind-the-scenes" way suit you better?
– Do you like interacting with other health care students and professionals or would you rather work more independently?

There are no right or wrong answers. These are simply preferences—a "wish list" of characteristics you have spontaneously spelled out. Just because you feel you would rather work in groups doesn't mean you will never work on your own. See Figure 3-1 for an example of a "wish list."

Did you try this exercise and end up with more blank paper than ideas? Are you struggling to differentiate between what you think you like and what mentors have said you should do? If you answered yes to either question, consider taking advantage of some type of personality assessment, such as the Myers-Briggs Type Indicator (MBTI), which helps you identify your preferred ways of perceiving the world and making decisions.

Myers-Briggs Type Indicator

The MBTI instrument, extrapolated from the theory of psychological types described by Swiss psychologist Carl Jung in the early 20th century, was designed during World War II to help women entering the industrial workforce identify war-time jobs where they would be "most comfortable and effective." The test, developed by Isabel Myers and her mother, Katharine Cook Briggs, is based on the concept that one's personality

Figure 3-1

Sample Wish List

Wish List
1. Patient interaction
2. Work as a member of a team
3. Opportunity for advancement
4. Opportunity to work on new & innovative projects
5. Time to devote to association involvement
6. Precepting opportunities
7. Didactic teaching opportunities
8. Good salary & benefits
9. Own desk, computer, + office space
10. East Coast Geography
11. Family-friendly work environment

type is similar to left- or right-handedness. We are each born with, or develop, preferred ways of thinking and acting. None of these ways is "better" or "worse," and your score on the test measures preferences, not aptitudes.

The instrument can give you insight into where you derive your energy, how you receive information, how you make decisions, and how you organize your personal world. Although it can be difficult for you to put the opposite psychological preferences into play—sort of like the discomfort right-handed people feel when trying to write their name with their left hand—you can become more proficient, and therefore more behaviorally flexible, with practice and development.

You are scored according to four "dichotomies," as shown in Table 3-1, each of which contains opposite preferences. Everyone uses all eight preferences to some degree, so your results are charted on a graph that shows the strength of your preferences. You receive a four-letter code showing which of the 16 different Myers-Briggs personality types describes you the best, based on your answers to the assessment instrument.

I, for example, am an ENTJ, which means I value organization and efficiency and tend to be very independent when making decisions. My extraversion is only slightly expressed, meaning that I probably have characteristics of both extraversion and introversion, depending on the situation. At times, I "recharge" by interacting with others in social situations, while at other times, being alone or in a small group is more relaxing. ENTJs tend to have a drive to learn new things on their own and are resourceful when solving problems. On the other hand, being an ENTJ means I'm not always comfortable with emotional or personal issues when compared with other personality types. In other words, the "touchy, feely" stuff isn't my favorite.

Table 3-1

The Myers-Briggs Type Indicator Dichotomies

Where a person focuses his or her attention	Extraversion (E)	Introversion (I)
	Tend to focus on the outer world of people and things	Tend to focus on the inner world of ideas and impressions
The way a person gathers information	Sensing (S)	Intuition (N)
	Tend to focus on the present and on concrete information gathered from their senses	Tend to focus on the future, with a view toward patterns and possibilities
The way a person makes decisions	Thinking (T)	Feeling (F)
	Tend to base decisions primarily on logic and objective analysis	Tend to base their decisions primarily on values and subjective evaluation of person-centered concerns
How a person deals with the outer world	Judging (J)	Perceiving (P)
	Tend to like a planned and organized approach to life and prefer to have things settled	Tend to like a flexible and spontaneous approach to life and prefer to keep options open

Adapted from: Hirsh SK, Kummerow JM. *Introduction to Type in Organizations*. 3rd ed. Mountain View, Calif: CPP, Inc.; 1998.

Classes on interpreting your MBTI and using it to improve your school or work life are available at many universities, particularly in schools of public health and career centers. For example, the University of North Carolina at Wilmington offers online access to the MBTI test for $11 per student, with the option to meet with a career counselor for further results interpretation. The University of North Carolina at Chapel Hill's School of Public Health offers a class titled "Using the Myers-Briggs Type Indicator to Build Teams across Disciplines" several times per year through the Office of Continuing Education. You can also look for assessment location options under the "Take the MBTI Instrument" section of the Myers & Briggs Foundation website at www.myersbriggs.org. Box 3-2 lists other sources of information on the MBTI.

Box 3-2

Sources of MBTI Information

Online

Assessments. If you can't find a class near you, take an online assessment at www.typefocus.com or www.humanmetrics.com.

Type Descriptions. For in-depth descriptions of the 16 types identified by the Myers-Briggs Type Indicator, visit www.typelogic.com or www.wikipedia.com.

Overall Information. Visit the Myers & Briggs Foundation website at www.myersbriggs.org or try some of the reading recommendations listed below.

Further Reading

On MBTI and Careers

Introduction to Type and Careers. Hammer AL. 1st ed. Palo Alto, Calif: Consulting Psychologists Press; 1993.

Looking at Type and Careers. Martin CR. 1st ed. Gainesville, Fla: Center for Applications of Psychological Type; 1995.

What's Your Type of Career? Unlock the Secrets of Your Personality to Find Your Perfect Career Path. Dunning D. 1st ed. Palo Alto, Calif: Davies-Black Publishing; 2001.

On MBTI Type in the Workplace

Introduction to Type in Organizations. Hirsh SK, Kummerow JM. 3rd ed. Mountain View, Calif: CPP, Inc.; 1998.

Looking at Type in the Workplace. Demarest L. 1st ed. Gainesville, Fla: Center for Applications of Psychological Type; 1997.

Type Talk at Work: *How the 16 Personality Types Determine Your Success on the Job*. Kroeger O, Thuesen JM. New York: Dell Publishing; 2002.

continued on page 27

Box 3-2

continued

Work It Out: Clues for Solving People Problems at Work. Hirsh SK, Kise JAG. 1st ed. Palo Alto, Calif: Davies-Black Publishing; 1996.

WorkTypes: Understanding Your Work Personality—How It Helps You and Holds You Back, and What You Can Do to Understand It. Kummerow JM, Barger NJ, Kirby L. 1st ed. New York: Warner Books; 1997.

On MBTI Type in Health Care

Health Care Communication Using Personality Type: Patients Are Different! Allen J, Brock SA. 1st ed. Hove, East Sussex, N.Y.: Routledge; 2003.

General MBTI References

Gifts Differing: Understanding Personality Type. Myers IB. Palo Alto, Calif: Davies-Black Publishing; 1995.

LifeKeys: Discover Who You Are. Kise JAG, Stark D, Hirsh SK. 2nd ed. Bloomington, Minn: Bethany House Publishing; 2005.

The 16 Personality Types: Descriptions for Self-Discovery. Berens LV, Nardi D. Huntington Beach, Calif: Telos Publications; 1999.

Type Talk: *The 16 Personality Types That Determine How We Live, Love, and Work*. Kroeger O, Thuesen JM. New York: Dell Publishing; 1989.

Was That Really Me? How Everyday Stress Brings Out Our Hidden Personality. Quenk NL. 1st ed. Palo Alto, Calif: Davies-Black Publishing; 2002.

Wired for Conflict: The Role of Personality in Resolving Differences. VanSant SS. 1st ed. Gainesville, Fla: Center for Applications of Psychological Type; 2003.

Work, Play, and Type: Achieving Balance in Your Life. Provost JA. 1st ed. Gainesville, Fla: Center for Applications of Psychological Type; 2001.

Resources for Choosing a Pharmacy Career Path

Of course, you can't make decisions about your career path in a vacuum. In addition to listing "likes" and "dislikes" and using tools such as the Myers-Briggs, you should take advantage of the many resources available to help you discover opportunities in the pharmacy profession.

Mentors and Advisors

Listen and learn from those around you. Fellow students, professors, advisors, friends, and family can all help you make the decision that is right for you.

I know, I know. Now you are completely confused. I just got through telling you to avoid being swayed by the opinions of others, and now I'm recommending that you get as much advice as you can find. What I mean is, seek advice but do not base your decisions solely on others' opinions. Take what you hear with a grain of salt and consider the source when evaluating information you are given.

For example, if you ask your preceptor, a clinical pharmacist specializing in pediatrics, for assistance in choosing a career path, she is likely to say that the best route is residency, specialization, and clinical patient care. And that may have been perfect for her, but it may not be right for you. Be sure to ask these questions:
- What do you like and dislike about your personal career path?
- What would you do differently if you could change something about your job?
- What experiences and training would you recommend for someone interested in a career like yours?

Remember, advice comes with biases. Consider each advisor's background, preferences, and personality type to help you frame their comments as best you can.

Networking

Learning how to network and make the most of contacts is important throughout your career, but at this stage, it can help you gain insights into several areas of pharmacy and get suggestions about the best fit for you.

Pharmacy is a small world. When a preceptor said that to me for the first time, I found it impossible to believe. I had to experience it to discover it's true—and the earlier you understand this and use it to your advantage, the better off you'll be.

Do you want to learn more about a career in transplant pharmacy? Mention your interest to a few mentors or professors, and you'll be surprised at the result. I've found it can play out like the "Six Degrees of Separation" game (for you *Footloose* fans—the "Six Degrees of Kevin Bacon" game). You're likely to hear, "I'm so glad you want to learn more about transplant pharmacy. Unfortunately, I forgot the little bit I learned years ago, but I happen to sit on a committee with an excellent transplant pharmacist. If you'd like, I can put you two in touch. I'm sure he wouldn't mind taking the time to tell you a little about his career path. I'll email him today!"

If you ask around, even in the informal way I just described, you'll be amazed at the resources and connections at your fingertips. Use these connections to your advantage, but make sure your inquiries are sincere and that you follow through. For example, if a preceptor puts you in touch with her colleague, it's your responsibility to connect and conduct yourself in a professional way. You are representing your preceptor when you interact with her colleague.

Be sure to let both pharmacists know how much you appreciate their assistance. Express your gratitude for the information and advice. Even if you decide after talking to the transplant pharmacist that you could never specialize in his area, he has helped you make an important discovery—and you can now cross that option off your list.

Professional meetings, such as the American Pharmacists Association (APhA) Annual Meeting, are a great place to network and explore career paths. Ask a preceptor or mentor to walk around with you and make introductions. You'll encounter pharmacists with a surprising range of expertise, and having met them at an association meeting makes it much easier to contact them in the future for assistance or advice.

I've found that pharmacists who participate in their associations, even if only by attending meetings, are usually very open to being approached by students. They understand how helping those coming up the ranks behind them benefits the profession.

Associations offer many resources to help you plan your career. A few are described in Box 3-3.

Box 3-3

A Sampling of Association-Based Resources for Career Planning

APhA Career Pathway Evaluation Program

(www.pharmacist.com)
One of the most comprehensive tools the American Pharmacists Association (APhA) offers is the Career Pathway Evaluation Program for Pharmacy Professionals, which helps you obtain knowledge about "two important subjects: the pharmacy profession and yourself," according to an introductory blurb on the APhA website. The program, which provides detailed pharmacy practice information and gives insights to help you choose the right career path, has four components:

— A briefing document and self-assessment exercises to complete before the workshop.
— A live workshop, lasting approximately two hours, provided by your school of pharmacy or a related organization.
— A workbook with materials and exercises to use during the live workshop.
— Follow-up exercises and resources to use after completing the workshop.

Most of the materials for the course can be located online at APhA's website, where you can take both written and online assessments and access all materials for the course. APhA trains facilitators for this workshop regularly; afterwards, they can hold

continued on page 30

Box 3-3

continued

workshops at their discretion. Although I never had the opportunity to participate in the live workshop, I learned a lot through the free online tools and assessments.

APhA Career Center

(www.pharmacist.com)
This online resource offers everything from assistance in building your résumé or curriculum vitae (CV) to a database of currently available jobs. Other features:
– Job alerts: Register for email notification when a new job is posted that meets your specifications.
– Résumé builder: Create a new professional résumé, tailored to highlight specific skills, or upload your existing résumé.
– Résumé databank: Post your résumé for maximum visibility with potential employers. This service gives you confidentiality while allowing employers to view your qualifications.
– Personalized websites: These password-protected websites include a home page, photo, references, and the ability to upload articles you've written or published.
– "My Work Style": A thorough, insightful survey that helps you learn ways to maximize your career success. It uncovers your work personality and matches your work style with various career paths.

ASHP's CareerPharm

(www.careerpharm.com)
The American Society of Health-System Pharmacists (ASHP) has an entire website to help pharmacists and students select and develop their careers, find jobs or residencies, and navigate the world of pharmacy practice.
– Highlights career profiles of pharmacists practicing in different areas of hospital and health-system practice.
– Provides tips on aspects of life as a pharmacist, including work-life balance, interviewing, and assessing salary and benefits packages.

ACCP Career Pathways

(www.accp.com/stunet/pathways.aspx)
The American College of Clinical Pharmacy (ACCP) offers the Career Pathways online compilation of profiles from active practitioners to help pharmacists, residents, and students explore their career goals.
– Profiles are organized by practice area for easy browsing and exploration.
– ACCP also offers career development tools such as interviewing tips, a directory of fellowships and residencies, and an online CV reviewing service, all of which are easily accessible from the same website.

Next Steps to Plan Your Destination

Pharmacy school teaches you excellent search skills you can apply to find many additional resources on your own. Use the tools described earlier in this chapter, and others you discover, to take action.

You can certainly put off deciding on a career path, but eventually you will end up working somewhere. The less proactive you are, the more likely you are to land in a career that is unrewarding for you.

When you get frustrated with the process of choosing a career path, remember the good news: more than one choice may be well suited to your likes, dislikes, and professional aspirations. You can have more than one "right answer."

For example, I enjoy providing direct patient care. However, my current job description as manager of outpatient pharmacy services at a regional hospital doesn't include much patient care. I was able to tweak the mission of our department to include a research component, and I now see patients as a part of a multinational clinical trial. Also, I've worked with a local psychologist to set up a mental health care service at our local free clinic, have obtained my prescribing license, and now see patients two nights per month in a direct patient care setting. The lesson? You can find ways to boost the success of your pharmacy setting while achieving your personal career goals.

Take out your list of "likes and dislikes" again. Now that you know more about yourself—based on the resources and assessments described in this chapter—you can create a scoring rubric to determine how well each career option you are considering matches your criteria. See Box 3-4 for instructions on creating such a rubric and Figure 3-2 for a sample rubric that might be used to assist in selecting a residency program. Box 3-5 provides a listing of further reading to help you learn more about specific pharmacy careers.

Although the rubric is a great way to objectify the career path selection process, in no way does it replace important subjective information you should consider. A career choice should not only look right on paper, it should *feel* right. As mentioned earlier, one of the best ways to obtain both the subjective and objective information you need about your potential career paths in pharmacy is to shadow or network with pharmacists practicing in those areas. While I can't possibly give you a comprehensive view of every career path in the profession of pharmacy, a few colleagues in a variety of roles agreed to tell you what you might expect if you were to walk a day in their shoes. See "A Day in the Life" on page 38.

Box 3-4

How to Make a Scoring Rubric

1. Review your notes on "likes and dislikes" to create a list of criteria important to you in your career.
2. Rank the items on your list in order of importance.
3. Give each item a weight, with the weights of all items totaling 100%.
4. Review potential pharmacy careers and list those that interest you the most. Be sure you understand the qualifications and additional training required for each career option you are considering.
5. Give each career option a score from 1 to 10, based on how well you think that career option would meet that criterion.
6. Multiply each score by the corresponding weight and tally the scores. The higher the score, the more closely that career path matches the criteria you selected.

Box 3-5

Further Reading on Pharmacy Careers

- **Community Pharmacy:** A Day in the Life of a Community Pharmacist. Masood A. *Student Pharmacist*. January/February 2007:12-5.
- **Federal Pharmacy:** Federal Pharmacy May Be the Best Career Secret. Schueller GH. *Pharmacy Student*. March/April 2004:20-2.
- **Managed Care:** Thinking of a Career in Managed Care Pharmacy? Flaherty J. *Pharmacy Student*. March/April 2005:30-1.
- **Nuclear Pharmacy:** Numerous Opportunities are Available in Nuclear Pharmacy. Vanderslice SD. *Pharmacy Student*. September/October 2003:20.
- **Pharmaceutical Industry:** Primed for an Industry Career. Mayer M. *Pharmacy Student*. November/December 2004:23.
- **Pharmacy Associations:** Association Work Offers Different View of Pharmacy Practice. Rochon J. *Pharmacy Student*. July/August 2003:24.
- **Pharmacy Law:** Combining Pharmacy and Law Provides Twice the Career Options. Bernstein IBG. *Pharmacy Student*. July/August 2003:16-7.
- **Transplant Pharmacy:** Are You Ready to Join the Transplant Critical Pharmacist Team? Eisenhart A. *Student Pharmacist*. January/February 2007:16-7.
- **Veterans Affairs Pharmacy:** VA Offers Advanced Practice Opportunities. Schueller GH. *Pharmacy Student*. May/June 2003:39.

Figure 3-2

Sample Rubric for Selecting a Career Path

Part 1. Criteria weighted by importance

Criterion	Work Hours	Vacation	Association Involvement	Precepting	Teaching	Patient Care	Geographic Area	Office Supplies & Equipment	Salary & Benefits	TOTAL
Weight	6%	4%	8%	10%	20%	30%	6%	8%	8%	100%
Career Type										
Career 1	2	1	8	4	8	6	5	5	4	
Career 2	8	5	7	6	7	9	9	7	6	
Career 3	9	8	5	5	4	8	6	9	5	
Career 4	4	6	6	8	6	5	7	6	2	
Career 5	6	1	4	2	2	7	5	3	1	

Part 2. Scoring for each criterion and career option

Criterion	Work Hours	Vacation	Association Involvement	Precepting	Teaching	Patient Care	Geographic Area	Office Supplies & Equipment	Salary & Benefits	TOTAL
Weight	6%	4%	8%	10%	20%	30%	6%	8%	8%	100%
Career Type										
Career 1	0.12	0.04	0.64	0.4	1.6	1.8	0.3	0.4	0.32	5.62
Career 2	0.48	0.2	0.56	0.6	1.4	2.7	0.54	0.56	0.48	7.52
Career 3	0.54	0.32	0.4	0.5	0.8	2.4	0.36	0.72	0.4	6.44
Career 4	0.24	0.24	0.48	0.8	1.2	1.5	0.42	0.48	0.16	5.52
Career 5	0.36	0.04	0.32	0.2	0.4	2.1	0.3	0.24	0.08	4.04

Explanation: In this sample rubric for scoring your career options, the top row in Part 1 contains a list of criteria, with each criterion weighted according to what this person considers most important. Then, each career type is given a score between 1 and 10 for each criterion, as shown in the main body of the table. Next, each score is multiplied by the respective weight, and the results are shown in Part 2. For example, Career 1 was given 2 out of 10 for "Work Hours"; after multiplying 2 by 0.06 (or 6%), the resulting number, 0.12, is plugged in. You complete the same process for each square in Part 1, fill in the numbers in Part 2, and add each career's score horizontally. As you can see, the mathematical "winner" is Career 2, but the applicant still needs to reflect on these results to determine if this career *feels* like the right fit.

Postgraduate Options

Some pharmacy careers call for postgraduate training. Postgraduate studies can also help you explore different pharmacy career paths. As stated in one postgraduate training opinion survey, "although the majority of postgraduate training appears to be residency-based, opportunities also exist for pharmacists to pursue fellowships, master's degrees, and even PhDs. These programs specialize in diverse settings, including basic, clinical, economic, social, and administrative sciences. Career plans of postgraduate students include employment in universities, the pharmaceutical industry, contract research firms, hospital and community pharmacy settings, and government organizations." You can even take part in dual degree programs in which you pursue two degrees simultaneously.

Dual Degree Programs

Because you earn two degrees at the same time—entry-level and advanced—dual degree programs save time and money while making you more marketable for certain types of positions, such as pharmacy administration, pharmaceutical research, or pharmacy law.

Dual degree programs, offered at many schools of pharmacy, vary widely in their focus and can give you opportunities to network and build skills in fields outside of pharmacy. Degrees that may be paired with the doctor of pharmacy curriculum include master of business administration (MBA), doctor of philosophy (PhD), master of science (MS), master of public health (MPH) and the juris doctor (JD). For more information about dual degree programs, I recommend reading the article "Dual Degrees in Pharmacy" by Marsha K. Millonig, published in the July/August 2003 issue of *Pharmacy Student*.

Residencies

The American Society of Health-System Pharmacists (ASHP) brochure, "Why Should I Do a Residency?" points out many reasons, "but the best have to do with learning how to apply the knowledge and skills you've learned in school to real patients, situations, and settings." Residencies give you hands-on experience and expose you to multiple career paths. According to ASHP, more than 1500 pharmacists complete residencies annually and there are more than 800 programs nationwide.

Each year, more and more pharmacy students undertake residencies to gain deeper experience before entering the job market. In fact, a survey by ASHP estimated that the number of residency programs more than doubled from 1996 to 2006, and placement of residents in programs has increased more than 10% annually every year since 2006. Some experts predict that eventually all prospective pharmacists—or at least those who provide direct patient care—will be expected to complete a residency as part of their professional training.

Residencies range from one-year pharmacy practice experiences to more advanced programs requiring several years to complete. The first year of the residency, called PGY1 year or postgraduate year 1, is designed to give you a general working knowledge of the area of practice in which you are training. PGY1 environments include hospitals, clinics, community practice, and managed care settings.

Many residency programs are accredited by ASHP and participate in the Resident Matching Program, commonly called "the Match," which is sponsored and supervised by ASHP. Accreditation assures prospective applicants that programs meet national quality standards. In addition, all accredited programs must take part in the Match process, which requires programs and prospective residents to follow the same timeline and process for applications, interviews, and candidate selections.

During the Match process, prospective residents apply to and interview with each residency program in which they are interested. After interviews are complete, candidates rank residency programs in order of preference while programs do the same with regard to their applicants. Residents and programs are then matched systematically to ensure that each program's and each resident's preferences are taken into consideration.

Unaccredited residency programs are also available, with their own application and interview process and a timeline that is typically similar to that of accredited programs—given that all programs recruit for their next class at approximately the same time of year. Unlike accredited programs, unaccredited residencies have not been surveyed and certified to meet certain quality criteria. They are also not subject to participation in the Match process and can use their own selection process and timeline.

When you finish a PGY1 residency program, you can choose to participate in a second year of residency, called the PGY2 or postgraduate year 2, which allows for study in a more focused area or "specialty" of the pharmacy profession. PGY2 programs also cover a variety of practice areas and interests, such as oncology, psychiatry, critical care, infectious disease, cardiology, and practice management, to name a few. Some PGY2 programs are also offered in conjunction with other degrees or fellowships, depending on the program.

For more information on residencies and a look at video vignettes providing an overview of residency programs, benefits to your career, and the residency selection process, visit the ASHP website at www.ashp.org. The resources provided at this site are comprehensive and even include a step-by-step walkthrough of the residency interview process, the Match, and the selection procedure. Click on Accreditation and choose Resident Information from the menu. Box 3-6 lists sources of additional information on residencies.

Box 3-6

Additional Information on Residencies

- Accelerate Your Career as a Resident. Burns A. *Pharmacy Student*. November/December 2004:9-11.
- APhA Foundation Executive Residency in Association Management & Leadership. Available at: www.aphafoundation.org/programs/The_Knowlton_Center.
- ASHP Online Residency Directory. Available at: accred.ashp.org/aps/pages/directory/residencyProgramSearch.aspx.
- ASHP Residency Information. Available at: www.ashp.org/Import/ACCREDITATION/ResidentInfo.aspx.
- Community Pharmacy Residency Program and Residency Locator. Available at: www.pharmacist.com/ResidencyLocator/ResidencyLocator.asp.
- The Hospital Residency Experience. Staggs SH. *Pharmacy Student*. November/December 2004:20.
- The Ins and Outs of the Residency Process. Ahrens R. *Pharmacy Student*. November/December 2004:12-4.
- What I Look For in a Resident. Weitzel K, Goad JA, Osterhaus M, et. al. *Pharmacy Student*. November/December 2004:24-5.

Advanced Graduate Studies

Advanced pharmaceutical studies come in many shapes and sizes. Pharmacists may choose to earn PhDs in medicinal chemistry, pharmaceutics, pharmacognosy, pharmacology, pharmacy administration, toxicology, and other areas of pharmacy. If such programs interest you, it's best to network with professors at schools of pharmacy or current PhD candidates to learn more.

At many schools of pharmacy, pharmaceutical companies, and other institutions, you can apply for fellowships to develop expertise in a specific type of scientific research, such as drug development, pharmacoeconomics, or pharmacokinetics. Fellowships are more focused on developing research skills whereas residencies are more focused on clinical skills. Fellowships tend to be highly individualized and require that you function as an independent investigator. In fact, many programs prefer for you to have completed at least one residency or obtained comparable clinical experience before applying for a fellowship. See Box 3-7 for more information on fellowships, or check the American College of Clinical Pharmacy website at www.accp.com.

Further Reading on Fellowships

Outcomes Research Fellowship

– A Burgeoning Opportunity for Future Pharmacists. Lee SP and Gagne JJ. *Student Pharmacist*. January/February 2007:19.

Pharmaceutical Industry Fellowships

– The Growth of Pharmaceutical Industry Fellowship Programs. Espinosa MG, Pao MS, Park PJ, et al. *Student Pharmacist*. January/February 2005:28-9.
– Pharmaceutical Fellowship Program Broadens Career Horizon. Burkhardt P, Lam AW, Patel K, et al. *Pharmacy Student*. January/February 2004:34.
– Soar Ever Higher in a Pharmaceutical Industry Fellowship. Shah C, Patel K, Shukla N, et al. *Student Pharmacist*. January/February 2007:22-3.

Is Extra Training Right for Me?

When deciding on a career path, think carefully about whether you want to—or will need to—pursue additional training. If you are considering four types of positions and three require residencies while one does not, you should seriously consider residency training. Additional training can also help you explore areas of interest and gain additional skills, which boosts your ability to find the right career for you.

Talk to people who are undergoing or have completed postgraduate training and ask lots of questions. For example:
– In your experience, what are the benefits of doing a residency?
– Why did you choose to pursue residency training in the first place?
– What criteria led you to the program you selected?

You should also ask your fellow pharmacy students about the advanced training they are considering, and why. Ask your professors and mentors which types of training they participated in and which they would recommend for you, based on your career goals.

Keep in mind that no matter which career or training choices you make, you'll need an effective curriculum vitae (CV), résumé, or both. The next chapter covers the basics for developing useful tools to market yourself.

A Day in the Life

Stories from Pharmacists in the Trenches

Clinical Coordinator
by Abbie Crisp Williamson, PharmD, BCPS

There really is no typical day for a clinical coordinator. Our role is similar to that of a clinical pharmacist with regard to direct patient care activities, but we also spend time in management and leadership. The ratio of time spent in direct patient care versus management activities depends on your specific job and institution. Below I've listed the typical day-to-day activities of a clinical coordinator based on two categories. Clinical coordinators must maintain the right balance of clinical, teaching, and direct patient care activities and of management and leadership activities to best meet the needs of their institution and staff.

Clinical, Teaching, and Direct Patient Care Activities
– Participating in patient care rounds
– Providing student and resident education
  • Rotation preceptor
  • Project preceptor
  • Presentation preceptor
  • Topic discussions
– Conducting research
– Providing in-service training
– Teaching didactic lectures
– Developing protocols and order sets
– Writing and submitting articles for publication

Management and Leadership Activities
– Scheduling staff
– Reviewing and approving time
– Running and attending staff meetings
– Planning staff development activities
– Evaluating performance
– Managing personnel
– Developing performance-improvement projects and initiatives
– Managing inventory
– Taking part in committees (internal and external)
– Maintaining involvement in professional organizations

7:00 am: Arrive to work; scan email for issues needing immediate attention—take action as needed.

7:30 am: Work up patients for patient care rounds.

8:00 am: Meet interdisciplinary team for patient care rounds.

10:00 am: Rounds end; check on clinical pharmacists staffing other services.

11:00 am: Participate in patient safety huddle.

11:30 am: Meet students to discuss assigned patients; develop pharmaco-therapy plan for each patient; follow-up or resolve patient care issues.

12:30 pm: Topic discussion with student pharmacists.

2:00 pm: Attend Pharmacy Leadership Team monthly meeting.

3:00 pm: Check and respond to email.

4:00 pm: Conduct area staff meeting.

5:00 pm: Type and post staff meeting minutes.

5:30 pm: Wrap up email; prepare for next day.

Public Health Emergency Preparedness Pharmacist
by Amanda F. Fuller, PharmD

What is an emergency preparedness pharmacist? Although the title varies, most states have a pharmacist charged with planning for pharmacy services during emergencies and disasters. Every day is different. The pharmacist is generally involved with the Strategic National Stockpile—medications and supplies maintained by the Centers for Disease Control and Prevention in case of a public health emergency—as well as with other federally funded pharmaceutical caches and state-level programs. Depending on the state, the public health emergency preparedness pharmacist may also work on communicable disease issues, be involved in managing state and national drug shortages, serve as a subject matter expert, participate in 24/7 on-call rotations, and work with legal counsel on developing and implementing state laws/rules.

24/7: Emergencies and disasters don't make appointments. They can happen anytime, so you never know when you might be called to duty. Events such as an anthrax release, a chemical or radiological release, a disease pandemic, or a hurricane require time and attention.

8:00 am: Arrive at the office to check overnight emails, voice mails, and the news. Follow up on any outstanding issues from the previous day's on-call log.

10:00 am: Put final touches on a continuing education (CE) presentation scheduled for tomorrow. Three to five CE programs or lectures are given every month to pharmacists and other health care providers on anything from anthrax to pandemic influenza.

11:00 am: Notify management of the call to the on-call pager reporting a suspicious substance being investigated in a county. Work with the county and public health partners to determine if prophylaxis is warranted and methods for carrying it out.

12:00 pm: Reschedule 3 pm meeting to plan for a press release related to antivirals used during the influenza pandemic.

1:00 pm: Continue work on state-level plans to dispense antibiotics or administer vaccinations to the state's 9.5 million residents.

3:00 pm: Meet with the state epidemiologist and other public health officials to develop and issue a press release.

4:30 pm: Return emails and voice mails from the day.

Pharmacy Coordinator for the Community Care of North Carolina Network
by Megan Rose, PharmD

Access III of the Lower Cape Fear, Inc., is a nonprofit partnership of primary care doctors, hospitals, county health departments, and county departments of social services. We are charged with improving health outcomes and reducing costs for residents of six counties who are enrolled in the state's low-income insurance plans. Fourteen networks, including ours, participate in the statewide Medicaid quality improvement strategy called Community Care of North Carolina (CCNC). We are involved in the following:

– Pharmacy Home Program for Medicaid patients with complicated medication regimens, in which we strive to increase medication adherence, decrease drug interactions, reduce unnecessary and duplicate medications, and improve patient outcomes.
– Medication therapy management services.
– Initiatives related to lists of approved prescription and nonprescription medications.
– Answering general medication questions.
– Providing education, including in-service training for providers and staff, group medical visits and presentations to patients, and brown bag medication reviews and counseling for patients.

8:00 am: Take part in conference call with pharmacists across the state to discuss initiatives regarding clinical, administrative, or e-prescribing matters.

9:00 am: Call pharmacies to clarify "Medicaid doesn't cover that" questions or to help patients secure medications.

10:00 am: Meeting with executive directors to discuss current and upcoming initiatives.

11:30 am: Home visit with patient recently discharged from hospital.

1:00 pm: Complete Medication Reconciliation/Medication Reviews for aged, blind, and disabled Medicaid patients admitted to hospitals in our six-county area.

2:00 pm: Attend Clinical Update/Education Meeting to prepare clinical training and education for our providers and case managers.

3:00 pm: Conduct medication reconciliation and reviews.

Pharmacy Association Director
by Ryan Swanson, PharmD

After four years of intense classroom education, countless disease state lectures, months of clinical rotations, and incalculable hours studying, very few pharmacy graduates find themselves in a career where they rarely—if ever—provide direct patient care. But these paths *do* exist, and I have discovered you can affect patients as much as when you work for a pharmacy association as you can by providing drug utilization reviews, counseling sessions, or medication reconciliations.

Nearly every state and national pharmacy association employs a pharmacist, from part-time grant writers to full-time executive directors. The population we deal with includes state legislators, dues-paying members, volunteer committee chairs, congressmen, lobbyists, and a public that often possesses very little knowledge of what pharmacists actually do. Our practice site isn't confined to four walls; it extends as far as our membership goes. And our goal? To advance the pharmacy profession.

8:30 am: Hold staff meeting regarding ongoing events and projects. With three continuing education programs coming up involving every staff person, it isn't difficult to overlook a vital aspect of any one meeting.

9:00 am: Call the association's lobbyist for an update on yesterday's late-night legislative budget hearings. There's always the chance, unfortunately, that pharmacy is being cut somewhere.

10:00 am: Review journal article ideas with the association's communications director. Settle on "Innovative Pharmacy Practices" as the next issue's theme.

10:30 am: Listen in on a conference call with the education counsel. Annual convention programming is nearly complete, although speakers for a "Medical Literature Update" session still need to be identified. Call three residency directors to recruit speakers.

11:15 am: Provide update at monthly Board of Pharmacy meeting on the activities of the association. Deliver the membership's consensus opinion on the mandatory counseling rule the Board has been considering.

12:00 pm: Attend working lunch with the chair of the association's newly formed Immunization Task Force, which has been charged with developing a proposal to expand pharmacists' immunization services in the state.

1:30 pm: Meet via a web-based session with student leaders from each of the state's schools of pharmacy to plan next semester's Student Leadership Conference.

3:00 pm: Draft grant requests for the association's annual meeting.

4:00 pm: Follow up on the day's questions from members, ranging from requests for missing CE certificates to offers to serve on the medication safety committee.

5:00 pm: On the way home, drop by a local pharmacy to say "hello" to a member pharmacist. The most effective association director is one who knows the people he represents and the professional issues they face.

Clinical Community Pharmacist
by Anthony T. Pudlo, PharmD, MBA

The amount of responsibility a clinical community pharmacist has in a traditional dispensing pharmacy depends on the demand for clinical pharmacy services within the community. We usually handle medication therapy management (MTM), disease state management, immunizations, and point-of-care screenings, and may find ourselves advocating for the growing role of the community pharmacist. Promoting a pharmacist's skill set to patients, physicians, insurance plans, employer groups, legislators, and even other pharmacists seems to be a daily occurrence. We are fully engaged in the community to foster health, wellness, and appropriate medication use. Those of us who work in well-established clinical community sites usually precept students on rotations and may even have a community pharmacy practice resident.

8:00 am: Arrive at work and participate in conference calls about updates in the community, such as health fairs, immunization protocols, or modifications to current MTM/disease state management programs.

8:30 am: Review patient charts or profiles for appointments scheduled for the day. Make sure administrative assistants, student pharmacists, and pharmacy residents understand their roles and responsibilities for the day.

9:00 am: Complete scheduled patient appointments, which may be phone-based or face-to-face. We also accommodate walk-in patients requesting immunization or point-of-care services.

12:00 pm: Meet with students and residents to review patient visits. Complete documentation and follow-up for patients seen in the morning. Have a topic discussion with students.

1:00 pm: Continue to meet with scheduled patients, who include those enrolled in formal disease state management, wellness, or education programs, such as those recognized by the American Diabetes Association or sponsored by employers. Continue immunization and point-of-care services for walk-in patients.

5:00 pm: Follow up on concerns from patients seen today or in the past. Review documentation and follow-up plans from students or residents.

6:00 pm: Leave for the day. Spend the evening catching up on new journal articles, preparing professional presentations, responding to emails, and working on personal research opportunities.

Clinical Staff Pharmacist on a Hospitalist Unit
by Jenna Reel, PharmD, BCPS

Pharmacists, either by training or genetics, tend to be detailed-oriented people. Other than that, there is no "typical" aspect for those of us serving as clinical staff pharmacists. We're involved in meetings, rounds, order entry, and instructional activities for pharmacy students and residents. I serve on the hospitalists' unit, working side-by-side with general practice physicians, assisting them in caring for their hospitalized patients.

8:00 am: Arrive at work and locate clinical notes left in the main pharmacy from nightshift staff that are relevant to the hospitalists' floor. Check on congestive heart failure (CHF) report, which is created for any patient admitted to the hospital within the last 24 hours with diagnosis of CHF. Don't forget pager.

8:30 am: Read emails and locate pneumonia patients admitted within the last 24 hours to hospitalists' floor, for the hospital's CMS Core Measures Initiative. (Many hospitals have a Core Measures Project, which helps to ensure that evidence-based, scientifically researched standards set by the Centers for Medicare & Medicaid Services [CMS] are followed when caring for patients.) Locate charts for patients admitted the day before and document that a chart review was performed and medications adjusted per patient's renal function.

9:00 am: Log onto computer and open work queues (Pyxis Connect) and order-entry queue (Meds Manager). Complete all consults requesting pharmacy to adjust medications for renal function. Complete all vancomycin, aminoglycoside, phenytoin, and other medication dosing requested by physician. Perform antibiotic streamlining on patients based on current culture and sensitivities.

Continue to perform order-entry tasks for the hospitalists' units.

11:00 am: Participate in interdisciplinary rounds.

12:00 pm: Meet with pharmacy students, residents, management, or pharmacy staff on various topics and eat lunch at the same time.

1:00 pm: Begin prospective chart reviews on all hospitalist patients admitted within the last 24 hours. Make recommendations and leave notes in charts. Follow up on recommendations made the previous days and update information in pharmacy computer system for further monitoring. Continue order-entry process for designated area.

3:00 pm: If a pharmacy student or resident is on rotation, review patients and follow up on questions they have pertaining to the patient's profile.

4:30 pm: Wrap up outstanding consults and pass to the clinical pharmacists any dose adjustments the physicians have requested. Head home, and after the little ones go to bed, review residents' and students' projects. Prepare for the next day.

Preparing Your Résumé, CV, and Portfolio

"Be selective in what you include on your résumé or CV, and present it in a concise, powerful way. Do not list every student presentation you've ever given. If you're still in school, your CV shouldn't be twice as long as a professor's."

—John P. Rovers, professor of pharmacy practice, Department of Pharmaceutical, Biomedical, and Administrative Sciences, Drake University

Laurie M. Whalin
2009 PharmD Recipient
Campbell University School of Pharmacy

We all know we need a professional résumé or curriculum vitae—and often, both—before securing a job or residency. But what exactly is the difference between a résumé and curriculum vitae? How should you go about preparing these vital career tools? And what is the role of a portfolio in your job search? This chapter will give helpful answers and serve as a quick reference. You'll also find additional resources in Box 4-1.

Box 4-1

Further Resources on Résumés and CVs

ACCP Online Curriculum Vitae Review Program
(www.accp.com/stunet/cv.aspx)
At this site you'll receive a helpful overview of how to prepare your curriculum vitae. You can also look at several sample CVs. If you're a student or postgraduate trainee and also a member of the American College of Clinical Pharmacy, you can submit your CV for review and editing by a volunteer ACCP reviewer.

ASHP's CareerPharm
(www.careerpharm.com)
From the CareerPharm homepage, a service of the American Society of Health-System Pharmacists, you can access information on writing CVs, résumés, cover letters, and thank-you correspondence. Tips from a pharmacy recruiter and information on "conquering the online job search" are also available under the "Resume, Curriculum Vitae (CV), and Cover Letter" dropdown.

continued on page 46

continued

Purdue Owl Online Writing Lab
(http://owl.english.purdue.edu/owl/resource/719/1)
This online resource gives tips for writing CVs, résumés, and cover letters and includes details such as page layout, choosing fonts, and proper ways to draw attention to items of interest. This web tool also provides information on preparing the content for your CV, résumé, and cover letter and gives samples of each.

The Pharmacy Professional's Guide to Résumés, CVs, & Interviewing
(Reinders TP. 2nd ed. Washington, D.C.: American Pharmacists Association; 2006.)
Inside this comprehensive guide, you'll find detailed instructions for developing your CV and résumé and nearly two dozen sample documents. It also covers interviewing, letters, and presenting a professional image.

The Résumé

A résumé is a brief summary of your education, professional history, and qualifications. Your résumé is meant to introduce you, briefly, to potential employers, so they are enticed to invite you for an in-person interview. A solid, strategically written résumé can make all the difference; it's a crucial marketing tool.

Your résumé should deliver a positive first impression and answer the question, "What skills and qualifications do you have that will be an asset to our company?" Your résumé can also serve as a reference during and after the interview process to prompt further questions about particular experiences or remind interviewers about your qualifications. The four key purposes of your résumé:
– A marketing brochure that emphasizes your skills and achievements.
– A calling card that briefly summarizes your experience.
– A reference document to help direct the interview.
– A reminder after the interview of who you are and what you bring to the position.

Résumé Formats

Résumés are typically no more than two pages long and follow one of four common formats, as explained in Box 4-2.

Box 4-2

Four Common Résumé Formats

Chronological	The most common type of résumé in pharmacy. Presents your work history in reverse chronological order for easy navigation.
Functional	Focuses more on your professional skills and de-emphasizes dates. Used most often by people changing careers or with gaps in their employment history.
Combination	Incorporates both a chronological and functional style to cover professional history, the skills you acquired, and your achievements during these experiences. This type of résumé is prevalent in most professions.
Targeted	Highly customized; this type of résumé specifically highlights your skills, experiences, and strengths that are relevant to the particular job you are applying for. Ideally, every résumé you submit when applying for an opportunity should be targeted, regardless of whether the résumé is chronological, functional, or a combination.

Guidebooks, career coaches, and other experts differ in their advice about what to include on your résumé, but some elements are universal. Below I'll explain the basic sections your résumé should contain.

Write your résumé in a direct, active, and concise style. Use short phrases instead of complete sentences, and avoid using the word "I," except in your career objective.

Contact Information

Your name should serve as the title to your résumé. Use your full name or your first name, middle initial, and last name and put it in a larger type size than all the other elements on your résumé. Include your address (both permanent and temporary addresses, if you're a student, with the dates you'll be at each), telephone number, and email address.

Remember, these are potential employers who'll be emailing or calling, so establish an appropriate email without embarrassing nicknames or phrases—not "sexigrl" or "surfdude." And make sure that the message on your voice mail is clear and professional.

You may also want to include in the contact information section on your résumé the URL of a professional social networking site where you have a presence, such as LinkedIn. (Found at www.linkedin.com, LinkedIn is an excellent place to post your qualifications online, network with contacts, and gather recommendations from people who can vouch for your skills and achievements.)

Career Objective

Including a career objective on your résumé is optional, but it can help hiring managers and others quickly grasp the focus of your job search. A well-written career objective helps establish your personal identity and emphasizes your main qualifications. You can think of it as akin to an advertising headline. Many people find writing a career objective to be the hardest part of creating a résumé.

When writing your career objective, avoid being too narrow or general. "To obtain a pharmacist position," is an example of an ineffective objective; it's far too vague and doesn't tell the reader anything useful. Try to communicate the type of position you want, the skills you offer, and your goals. Below are some sample objectives.

- "To obtain a pharmacy internship position where I can apply my clinical knowledge and enhance my skills to prepare for a career as a clinical pharmacist."
- "To join a health-system pharmacy where I can apply my knowledge and expertise as a drug information specialist."

Education

List in reverse chronological order your educational experiences, including name of institution, dates attended, degree obtained, and major or concentration. Optional information you may want to include is relevant coursework, research or thesis work, and honors received.

If you're a student or new graduate, list your education before your experience, because it's likely to be the most relevant link to the position you're seeking. Once you have more professional experience under your belt, put that section before education.

Experience

List in reverse chronological order your professional experiences including position held, name and location of institution, and dates of service. Then include a brief description of your work that focuses on responsibilities demonstrating initiative, transferable skills, and results. Choose energetic action verbs to describe your activities, such as those listed in Box 4-3, because they present your skills and accomplishments in a powerful way. When potential employers scan résumés, they are looking for evidence that you will enhance the workplace and help solve problems—not merely go through the motions to complete a task.

Box 4-3

A Sampling of Action Verbs

Achieved	Created	Exceeded	Organized
Adapted	Cut	Expanded	Prepared
Advanced	Defined	Formulated	Presented
Analyzed	Delivered	Generated	Prevented
Attained	Demonstrated	Guided	Produced
Budgeted	Designed	Identified	Reduced
Built	Detected	Improved	Resolved
Calculated	Developed	Increased	Saved
Centralized	Devised	Initiated	Secured
Chaired	Directed	Investigated	Simplified
Charted	Discovered	Launched	Standardized
Changed	Enabled	Led	Supervised
Compiled	Enacted	Managed	Trained
Conducted	Enforced	Measured	Upgraded
Converted	Enhanced	Motivated	
Counseled	Established	Negotiated	

Today, professional career coaches advise job candidates in all professions to emphasize achievements on their résumés. A simple way to do this is to think of key actions you carried out in a position and link each with a benefit. For example, instead of simply saying, "organized student association meetings," ask yourself, "so what?" to think of a compelling way to finish the statement. The result might be "organized student association meetings to ensure that major projects and fundraisers were accomplished on schedule." Box 4-4 gives a few more examples.

Box 4-4

Sample Statements for Emphasizing Achievements on Résumés

Action	Benefit
Processed prescription insurance claims	to improve accuracy and timely payment
Counseled patients about proper use of medications	to promote compliance and prevent adverse effects

Memberships, Service, and Leadership

Include memberships, service roles, and leadership activities, particularly those related to college, your community, and pharmacy or health care. List years of service, positions you held, and specific recognition gained. This section helps future employers recognize that you are well rounded and possess initiative and motivation.

Awards and Honors

List brief information about awards, accolades, and honors you have received, particularly those relevant to the position you're seeking.

References

Do not include references on your résumé. Instead, compile a separate reference sheet with the names, titles, and contact information of people who can vouch for your skills, experience, and contributions in case a potential employer requests reference information before or during an interview. Some people include the statement, "References available on request," but it's unnecessary to say this on your résumé.

Optional Sections

You can create other sections on your résumé, depending on your background and the type of position you are seeking. For example, you might include such headings as licenses and certificates, committees, research interests, publications and presentations, or special skills and training. Figures 4-1 and 4-2 show sample résumés.

The Curriculum Vitae

The curriculum vitae, or CV, differs most notably from a résumé in its length. Résumés are limited to one or two pages, while CVs for most professionals are typically three or more pages long. CVs are comprehensive documents used in such fields as academia, health care, law, and engineering to provide details about professional background, education, qualifications, and experiences.

A CV is a living document that is updated frequently to reflect ongoing developments in your career. Most pharmacists prepare both a résumé and a curriculum vitae, because they serve different purposes. You use your résumé, which gives a brief snapshot of your qualifications, when applying for specific positions—it's a marketing document. Your CV, on the other hand, is informational. You use it when applying for postgraduate residencies or fellowships, seeking academic and organizational leadership positions, or entering the nomination process for honors and awards.

CVs do not follow a universal format the way résumés do, and because length is not restricted, you are free to include additional categories and subheads reflecting your

Figure 4-1

One-Page Résumé for Pharmacy Intern

Timothy P. Gonzalez

<u>Local Address</u>	<u>Permanent Address</u>
4029 Edgewood Road	2039 West Long Street
Chapel Hill, North Carolina 03948	Rockville, Maryland 30495
(927) 924-7593	(917) 728-9803
Email: tpgonzalez@email.unc.edu	

OBJECTIVE: Pharmacy intern position in a community pharmacy where I can apply and enhance my customer service skills, knowledge of pharmacy practice, and pharmacy terminology.

EDUCATION:

University of North Carolina at Chapel Hill   August 2006–Present
Chapel Hill, North Carolina   Anticipated Graduation: 2010
Major: Chemistry   G.P.A.: 3.4 / 4.0

West Rockville High School   September 2002–May 2006
Rockville, Maryland

EXPERIENCE:

Receptionist, Langley Law Firm   June 2006–August 2006
Rockville, Maryland
Achievements: Received award
for exceptional customer relations

Sales Associate, Tanya's Formalwear   May 2005–August 2005
Scottsville, Arizona
Achievements: Developed flyers, coupons, and
special promotions to boost prom season business

Lifeguard, Rockville Country Club   June 2003–August 2003
Rockville, Maryland
Achievements: Planned/taught water aerobics class
for senior citizens 3 days/week to improve cardiovascular
fitness and promote exercise as fun and healthy

Volunteer, Saint Mary Hospital   July 2002–December 2005
Rockville, Maryland
(4–20 Hours/Week)
Achievements: Spent 4-20 hours/week orienting patients
and families to hospital services and developed special
handout to answer their key questions

CERTIFICATES:

American Red Cross Adult CPR Certificate   2001–Present
American Red Cross First Aid Certificate   2001–2005
American Red Cross Infant & Child CPR   2001–2005

MEMBERSHIPS:

Student Member, UNC Alumni Association   2006–Present
Chemistry Club, University of North Carolina   2006–Present

LANGUAGES:

Fluent in English and Spanish

Figure 4-2

Two-Page Résumé for Pharmacy Intern

Christina R. Alexander

8372 Bay Street
Charleston, South Carolina 29401

Telephone: 928.766.2004
Email: calexander12@aol.com

CAREER OBJECTIVE

To obtain a pharmacy internship that enhances my strengths, expands my knowledge, and allows me to contribute my skills to further the organization's goals.

PROFESSIONAL SUMMARY

Pharmacy intern with excellent communication, leadership, and organizational skills. Background in research, patient education, and pharmacy practice.

EDUCATION

Medical University of South Carolina
School of Pharmacy
Charleston, South Carolina

2006–Present
Degree anticipated May 2010

University of Virginia
Charlottesville, Virginia

2002–2006
B.S. in Biology

PROFESSIONAL EXPERIENCE

Pharmacy Technician, St. Mark's Medical Center
Charleston, South Carolina

2007–Present
(Part-time)

- Conducted study with over 100 participants, comparing effectiveness of web-based tools to communicate information about drug therapy

- Organized and updated records from pharmacists' patient counseling sessions

- Presented information sessions on home medication safety for parents of young children

- Organized and participated in quarterly monthly "brown bag" sessions on behalf of the medical center at a local senior center in which pharmacists reviewed medication profiles of seniors

Figure 4-2

continued

Christina R. Alexander   Page 2

PROFESSIONAL EXPERIENCE (Continued)

Pharmacy Technician, Seahorse Drugs   2006–2007
Charleston, South Carolina   (Summer)

- Obtained, organized, and displayed educational materials for patients with chronic diseases, including asthma, diabetes, allergies, and osteoporosis

- Evaluated options for updating telephone system to make requesting prescription refills easier for patients

- Collaborated with two other technicians to publish a monthly wellness newsletter

Laboratory Assistant I   2004–2005
Biology Department   (Summer)
University of Virginia

- Inventoried and reordered supplies and maintained stock records for department chair

- Mentored students in two sections of Introduction to Biology summer course

MEMBERSHIPS

American Pharmacists Association   2006–Present
  Academy of Student Pharmacists (APhA-ASP)
South Carolina Association of Pharmacy Students   2006–Present

AWARDS AND HONORS

APhA-ASP Chapter Vice President   2008

Chair, Operation Diabetes Campaign   2008
  Promoting early screening and detection

Poster Presentation, Diabetes Awareness   2008
  APhA-ASP Meeting

Service Award, Taking Action by Service, for planning and   2007
  implementing a high school science tutoring program

Psi Theta Mu National Biological Honor Society   2005–2006

Dean's List, College of Arts and Sciences   2002–2006
University of Virginia

personal and professional experiences. However, most disciplines have adopted conventions for emphasizing particular points on the CV that are relevant to that profession. To become familiar with these conventions, look at CV examples from your preceptors and mentors and from other people in the pharmacy profession. Chapter 10 contains useful guidelines for how to keep your CV updated and adapt it for specific uses. Always keep one comprehensive version as a master, but tailor the ones you use for specific purposes so the most relevant publications, presentations, and activities are included.

Personal Information

The words "Curriculum Vitae" serve as the title of your document and should appear at the top of the first page, centered. Below that, list your personal information: full name, address (temporary and permanent), phone number, and email address. Some people choose to place this information under the heading "Personal Information," but it's really a matter of your preference.

Career Objective

According to Thomas Reinders, author of *The Pharmacy Professional's Guide to Résumés, CVs, & Interviewing,* most pharmacists and health professionals do not include a career objective on their CV. In cases where you can't or don't submit a cover letter, however, a statement about your career objective, similar to the ones on page 48, may be your only chance to introduce yourself and highlight your skills and qualifications.

Educational Experience

List in reverse chronological order your educational experiences, including name of institution, dates attended, degree obtained, and major or concentration. In a CV, it's standard to include relevant coursework that is not be reflected in your degree, as well as any research or thesis work.

Giving your academic standing is optional, but Reinders recommends including it if you are applying for a residency or fellowship. You can present your academic standing by using grade point average—in a format that conveys your school's scale, such as 3.5/4.0; by class ranking; or by stating your graduation honors (cum laude).

Professional Training

Consider including a section titled "Professional Training" if you've completed a post-graduate residency or fellowship. You can also include that information under the education or professional experience sections, but you run the risk of potential employers overlooking it. By adding a separate heading, you can be sure to draw attention to your specialized training. Give the name and location of the institution, the dates attended, and the type of certification you earned.

Professional Experience

As in the educational experience section, list in reverse chronological order your professional experiences, including position held, name and location of institution, and dates of service. Also include a description of your work, focusing on responsibilities that demonstrate initiative, transferable skills, and results. Use action verbs, such as the examples in Box 4-3. You can put volunteer experience here if it was a long-term commitment and it allowed you to use your professional knowledge and abilities.

Research Experience

Briefly describe your undergraduate, doctoral, and postdoctoral research endeavors, including projects, grants, and patents. List them in reverse chronological order and include title, name of sponsoring agency or institution, co-investigators, dates, and outcomes. It's also helpful to give descriptions of any specific contributions you made.

Teaching Experience

Placing your teaching experience and faculty appointments under a separate heading helps emphasize these qualifications. If you wish, however, you can include them in the "Professional Experience" section. List the institution, course number and title if available, the date, your title (lecturer, teaching fellow, resident), and number of students involved.

Publications and Presentations

You can combine these categories under one header or present them as two separate categories, depending on how many samples you'll be listing. Types of publications you should include are books, abstracts, articles, and reviews you have written. If you have a substantial number of each, consider grouping them under subheadings. Follow appropriate citation forms, such as the approach presented in the *American Medical Association Manual of Style,* and remember to be consistent throughout your CV.

List presentations in reverse chronological order and include the title of your presentation, the institution or organization either sponsoring it or hosting it, date, location, and your audience.

Licensure and Certifications

List the types of licenses and certifications you hold, including the awarding agency, full title of the license or certificate, license/certificate number, date issued, and renewal date. Types of certificates often listed by pharmacy professionals on their CVs include:
- Basic life support (BLS) or advanced cardiac life support (ACLS)
- Board of Pharmacy Specialties designations such as BCPS (Board Certified Pharmacotherapy Specialist)

- Accreditation Council for Pharmacy Education (ACPE) certificates
- Residency certificates

Awards and Honors

Present your awards or honors in reverse chronological order and include the name or title of the award, sponsoring agency or institution, location where the award was given, and the date you received it.

Professional Memberships

Listing memberships in professional organizations highlights your dedication to the profession of pharmacy. Include the name of the organization, the dates during which you were a member, and any offices held, task force appointments, or activities you participated in. Thomas Reinders suggests including an additional heading called "Leadership Experience" if you've participated extensively in professional organizations, because it allows you to emphasize your role and elaborate on your involvement.

Service Activities

In this section you can include volunteer work, community service activities, or university committees you participated in. You don't want to keep repeating items on your CV however, so if you listed an office you held in a professional organization under "Professional Memberships," don't include it in the service activities section too.

References

The advice about not including reference names and contact information on your résumé also applies to CVs. Instead, create a separate reference page you can quickly supply if requested. Be sure to notify your references beforehand that you will be listing them, and always provide them with the most updated copy of your CV.

Optional Sections

Depending on your background, sections you might include on your CV include military service, scholarly associations, study abroad, or other work experience. Figure 4-3 provides an example of a CV.

The Portfolio

A professional portfolio is a great way to showcase your professional experience, growth, and achievements in a way that's not possible in a traditional résumé or curriculum vitae. Portfolios are visual, helping the reader relate to you in a tangible way, and they contain details you can't pack into a résumé. Today many schools of pharmacy encourage and even require students to develop a portfolio before they graduate.

Figure 4-3

CV for Pharmacy Resident

Curriculum Vitae

DALLAS MONTGOMERY

123 Main Street
Wilmington, NC 28415
910-373-4441
dmontgomery@webmail.com

EDUCATION

Primary Care Specialty Residency
New Hanover Regional Medical Center
Wilmington, N.C.   *July 2009–Present*
- *Residency Director: Bruce Canaday, PharmD, BCPS*

Doctor of Pharmacy
University of North Carolina at Chapel Hill   *2005–2009*
- Degree received May 2009

Bachelor of Science in Biology
University of North Carolina at Chapel Hill   *2002–2005*
- Minor in Chemistry
- Degree received May 2006

TRAINING

Spanish for Healthcare Professionals
   Coastal AHEC Continuing Education   *March–May 2010*

ACCP Heart Failure Training Program
American College of Clinical Pharmacy & UNC Hospitals   *February 2010*
- *Preceptor: Herbert Patterson, PharmD*

PROFESSIONAL ORGANIZATIONS

New Hanover Regional Medical Center   *2009–Present*
   Antibiotic Subcommittee
   Pharmacy & Therapeutics Committee
    Secretary *(2009– 2010)*

American College of Clinical Pharmacy   *2009–Present*
   Associate Member in Training

FIP (International Pharmaceutical Federation)   *2009–Present*
   Community Pharmacy Section
   Young Pharmacists' Group

UNC School of Pharmacy Student Government   *2008–Present*
   PY4 Class Vice-President *(2008–2009)*

Kappa Epsilon Fraternity   *2007–Present*
Pledge Class Social Committee Chair *(Fall 2007)*
Fundraising and Service Committees *(2007)*

Figure 4-3

continued

APhA (American Pharmacists Association)   *2005–Present*
New Practitioner Initiative Web Site Task Force *(2009–2010)*

ASHP (American Society of Health-System Pharmacists)   *2005–Present*
New Practitioners Forum
     Forum Vice-Chair *(June 2008–June 2009)*
     Web Site Focus Group *(June 2009)*
     Exhibitor at the Southeastern Residency Conference *(May 2008)*
     Leadership and Career Development Subcommittee *(January–June 2005)*

CAPS (Carolina Association of Pharmacy Students)   *2005–2009*
Executive Committee Member *(2007–2008)*

IPSF (International Pharmaceutical Students' Federation)   *2005–2009*
UNC School of Pharmacy Liaison *(2007–2008)*

HONORS, AWARDS, & CERTIFICATIONS

Coastal AHEC Internal Medicine Scholarly Achievement Award   *2010*
Advanced Cardiac Life Support Certification   *2009*
Facts and Comparisons Excellence in Clinical Communications Award   *2009*
Phi Lambda Sigma Leadership Society   *2008–Present*
1st Place, ASHP National Clinical Skills Competition   *2008*
UNC School of Pharmacy Graduation Marshall   *2008*
APhA Immunization Certification   *2007*

PUBLICATIONS

Montgomery D. Journal club 101 for the new practitioner: Evaluation of a clinical trial. *Am J Health-Syst Pharm.* 2010;61:1885-6.

Montgomery D. Tips on Opening Your Own Pharmacy. *Transitions: A Communication for APhA New Practitioners.* Spring 2010.

POSTERS

Hormone Replacement Therapy Subsequent to the Women's Health Initiative
Primary Care Residency Project
• American College of Clinical Pharmacy Annual Meeting   *October 2009*
• Coastal AHEC Research Day   *June 2009*
• 2010 Southeastern Residency Conference   *May 2009*

Implementation of a Dofetilide Order Sheet in a Community Hospital Setting
American College of Clinical Pharmacy
• Annual Meeting Cardiology Poster Session   *November 2008*

Figure 4-3

continued

Dallas Montgomery   Page 3 of 6

PRESENTATIONS

Spiriva (tiotropium)
Formulary Review   *April 2010*
- Presented to NHRMC Pharmacy & Therapeutics Committee

Pain Management for the Family Medicine Resident
Disease State Management Presentation   *March 2010*
- Presented to Coastal Family Medicine faculty, students, and residents

Peripartum Cardiomyopathy
Patient Case Presentation   *February 2010*
- Presented to UNC Heart Center faculty and trainees

Guidelines for the Management of Chronic Heart Failure
Guidelines Presentation   *January 2010–April 2010*
- Presented to Coastal Family Medicine faculty, residents, and students
- Presented to Coastal AHEC faculty, residents, and students
- Pharmacy Staff Inservice

**Guidelines for the Use of Antiretroviral Agents in
HIV-1-Infected Adults and Adolescents**
Guidelines Presentation   *December 2009–April 2010*
- Presented to Coastal AHEC faculty & students
- Pharmacy Staff Inservice
- Coastal AHEC Pharmacist Continuing Education Course

Emend (aprepitant)
Formulary Review   *October 2009*
- Presented to NHRMC Pharmacy & Therapeutics Committee

Fuzeon (enfuvirtide)
New Drug Monograph Presentation   *April 2009*
- Presented to faculty, residents, and students of Coastal AHEC

Atrial Fibrillation: Rhythm Control versus Rate Control
Journal Club Presentation   *February 2009*
- Presented to faculty, residents, and students of Coastal AHEC

Use of Nonsteroidal Antiandrogens in the Treatment of Prostate Cancer
Patient Care Presentation   *November 2008*
- Presented to faculty, residents, and students of Coastal AHEC

Osteoporosis
Ambulatory Care Presentation   *August 2008*
- Presented to faculty and residents of Coastal AHEC

Pfizer and Viagra: A Love Story
Pharmaceutical Research, Development, and Marketing Presentation   *Fall 2007*
- Presented to faculty and students of UNC School of Pharmacy
and UNC School of Business

Echinacea
Herbal Products Presentation   *Spring 2006*
- Presented to faculty and students of UNC School of Pharmacy

Figure 4-3

continued

Dallas Montgomery	Page 4 of 6

PROJECTS

Pharmagram: A Newsletter for Health Care Professionals
Staff writer of bimonthly newsletter *2008–Present*
• New Hanover Regional Medical Center

Revisiting a Retrospective Evaluation of Vitamin K Use in Medical/Surgical Patients
Medication Utilization Evaluation *April 2010*
• New Hanover Regional Medical Center

Hyponatremia Protocol
Protocol for the treatment of hyponatremia in an inpatient setting *March 2010*
• New Hanover Regional Medical Center

Obstetrics Rotation Background Reading Coursebook
Developed a collection of background readings for future residents *February 2010*
pursuing the Complicated Obstetrics Rotation
• New Hanover Regional Medical Center

Oral Contraceptives
Therapeutic Class Review *January 2010*
• Coastal Family Medicine

Primary Care Residency Manual
Organized and developed the residency manual for the Primary *December 2009*
Care Residency Program
• New Hanover Regional Medical Center

Alcohol Withdrawal Drug Utilization Evaluation
Retrospective chart review of alcohol withdrawal treatment at *January 2009*
Mission St. Joseph's Hospital
• Substance Abuse, Mountain AHEC

Direct to Consumer Advertising
Ethical Dilemma Project *April 2008*
• UNC School of Pharmacy

COX-II Drug Utilization Evaluation Form
DUE Data Collection Form & Protocol *October 2007*
• UNC School of Pharmacy

OTC Formulary Handbook
Pocket reference for community pharmacists *November 2007*
• UNC School of Pharmacy

LEADERSHIP AND SERVICE ACTIVITIES

SMAT-II Disaster Response Team
Steering Committee *2005–Present*
Volunteer Pharmacist and Clinician *2009–Present*

Figure 4-3

continued

Tileston Outreach Health Center
Health Care Clinic Pharmacy Volunteer   *2009–Present*

Health for Habitat
Steering Committee   *2007–2008*

Taking Action by Service
Interfaith Council Homeless Shelter Volunteer   *2007–2008*
Meals on Wheels Volunteer   *2007–2008*
Relay for Life Volunteer   *2007–2008*
Ronald McDonald House Volunteer   *2007–2008*
UNC Children's Hospital Volunteer   *2007–2008*

IPSF (International Pharmaceutical Students' Federation)
Book Drive Chairperson   *Fall 2007*

RESIDENCY ROTATIONS

Ambulatory Care & HIV Rotation (Longitudinal)
New Hanover Regional Medical Center   *May 15–Present*
Wilmington, N.C.
Preceptor: Kim Thrasher, PharmD, BCPS

Psychology Rotation
Coastal Family Medicine & Coastal Horizons Center   *May 3–14, 2010*
Wilmington, N.C.
Preceptor: Lisa Easterling, PharmD

Outpatient HIV Clinic Rotation
New Hanover Regional Medical Center   *April 2010*
Wilmington, N.C.
Preceptor: Kim Thrasher, PharmD, BCPS

Complicated Obstetrics Rotation
New Hanover Regional Medical Center   *March 2010*
Wilmington, N.C.
Preceptor: Kim Thrasher, PharmD, BCPS

ACCP Heart Failure Traineeship
University of North Carolina Heart Failure Program   *February 2010*
Chapel Hill, N.C.
Preceptor: Herbert Patterson, BS, PharmD

Family Medicine Rotation
Coastal Family Medicine   *December 2009–January 2010*
Wilmington, N.C.
Preceptor: Lisa Easterling, PharmD

Figure 4-3

continued

Ambulatory Care Rotation
New Hanover Regional Medical Center   *October–November 2009*
Wilmington, N.C.
Preceptor: Kim Thrasher, PharmD, BCPS

Internal Medicine Rotation
New Hanover Regional Medical Center   *July–August 2009*
Wilmington, N.C.
Preceptor: Bruce Canaday, PharmD, BCPS

Pharmacy Practice Rotation
New Hanover Regional Medical Center   *June 2009*
Wilmington, N.C.
Preceptor: Larry Hovis, RPh

EMPLOYMENT

Trade & Pharmacy Affairs Intern
GlaxoSmithKline, Philadelphia, Pa.   *May–July 2008*
Preceptor: Stephen J. Kalinowski, RPh
• Wrote medical letters, positioning and mission statements, and pharmacy organization
correspondence; managed projects for product teams; developed content for trade and pharmacy
affairs initiatives, brand team strategies, and managerial programs for pharmacy leaders;
created presentations and launch materials for GSK/Bayer sales force, regional sales trainers,
and account managers; and supported trade and pharmacy objectives to ensure appropriate
distribution, stocking, and wholesaler/chain interaction for launch products, line extensions,
and current products.

Student Intern
Eckerd Pharmacy, Raleigh, N.C.   *Summer 2007*
Preceptor: Wes Cotton, RPh
• Filled prescriptions, counseled patients, entered computer system information, applied
for patient insurance reimbursements, completed order requests, participated in a recall
program, received telephone prescription orders from physicians' offices, applied and
expanded drug information knowledge and computer skills.

Pharmacy Technician
CVS Pharmacy, Chapel Hill, N.C.   *Summer 2006*
Preceptor: Wes Sutton, RPh
• Filled prescriptions, counseled patients, restocked shelves, entered computer system
information, developed brand/generic and drug information knowledge, honed communi-
cation skills.

SPECIAL SKILLS

Web Page Design (including HTML and basic JavaScript)
Microsoft Word, PowerPoint, Excel, and Access
Spanish Language

Through a professional portfolio, you can display materials related to your work and accomplishments as you progress through your career—presenting evidence of how far you've come and where you're headed in the future. The portfolio format should be businesslike and should include an outline of the information contained within your portfolio so it's easy for the reader to navigate. Boxes 4-5 and 4-6 provide sample tables of contents for two different portfolios.

Box 4-5

Sample Table of Contents for a Residency Portfolio

Professional Development
Quarterly Review
Curriculum Vitae
Goals
CE & Certificates

Pharmacy Department
Formulary Review
P & T Minutes
Pharmacy Newsletter Articles

Student Seminar
Presentations

Research
Residency Project
Drug Utilization Review
Poster Project

Presentations (List these by title)
Presentation #1
Presentation #2
Presentation #3
Presentation #4
Presentation #5

Projects (List these by title)
Project #1
Project #2
Project #3
Project #4

Patient Care & Intervention
Sample Notes: Ambulatory Care
Sample Notes: Family Medicine
Sample Notes: Inpatient Medicine

Evaluation
Quarterly
Mid-Point
Final Site/Preceptor Evaluation
Self Evaluation

Thanks to the technological world we live in, portfolios can be electronic—either in a CD-ROM format or maintained on the Internet for easy access. Even so, many students and recent graduates prefer to maintain "hard-copy" portfolios they can bring with them on interviews. These types of portfolios should be created in a clean, plain, three-ring binder (see Figure 4-4 for examples). The sections described below are commonly included in portfolios. Personally, I bring a copy of my portfolio to every interview and offer it as an example of my previous work and achievements. If the interviewer declines my offer to review this information, I simply tuck it away in my attaché. Although many interviewers will not request a portfolio, you'll be surprised how many will want to review it if you bring it along.

Box 4-6

Sample Table of Contents for a Professional Portfolio

Curriculum Vitae

Goals

Continuing Education

Honors and Awards

Press

Positions

Publications

Presentations (List these by title)
> Presentation #1
> Presentation #2
> Presentation #3
> Presentation #4
> Presentation #5

Projects (List these by title)
> Project #1
> Project #2
> Project #3
> Project #4

Maintaining a portfolio is also a great way to keep your CV or résumé up to date. After I give a formal presentation, I put a copy of my PowerPoint slides in a folder called "To Add to CV and Portfolio." Periodically, I take out this folder, add the names of presentations and other documents to my CV, cover the hard-copy material with plastic page covers, and place it in my portfolio. Of course, there will always be items in your portfolio that are not referenced by your CV or résumé, and vice versa, but developing a process for updating everything simultaneously can ensure that you don't omit any important information.

Figure 4-4

Examples of Portfolio Binders

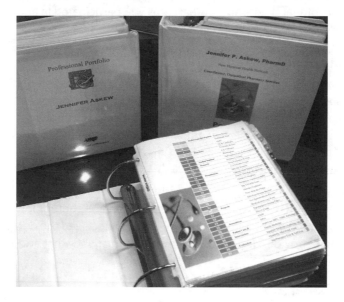

I recommend that you keep a separate portfolio for each major learning program, such as pharmacy school, a residency, or a fellowship. I have both a Student Portfolio and a Residency Portfolio. Later, I will have one Professional Portfolio until it becomes cumbersome in size. Then I'll thin it out or separate it into binders for certain time frames, such as each year, two years, or five years of practice.

Personal Information

Place either your résumé or your curriculum vitae, which supplies all your contact information, at the beginning of your portfolio. If you choose, you can include additional personal information, such as:

- Photograph of yourself.
- Personal statement reflecting your career goals.
- Statement of your professional philosophy (your practice philosophy, for example, or your philosophy related to teaching or research, if relevant).
- Personal interests.

Education

You can create a separate section for education to list the universities you attended, along with the degrees you obtained from each. Include a copy of your diplomas as well as descriptions, outlines, or examples of thesis work or research you completed at each university.

Experiential Learning

If you are a new graduate or have recently completed a residency, list your rotations along with the site and preceptor information. Include copies of evaluations from your preceptor and note any journal clubs you participated in and projects or presentations you completed during that rotation.

Awards and Honors

Present the names and a brief description of awards, honors, or recognition you've received. If possible, include a copy of the award, if it was a certificate. Or you can put in a photograph of the actual award, or of you receiving the award, which adds a personal touch and helps the viewer visually connect you to the award.

Licensure and Certifications

In this section, list the individual licenses and certifications you've obtained, including a brief description of each. Incorporate photocopies or photographs of the actual documents if you can. Another option, if you have not received the document yet, for example, is to provide a letter from the accrediting agency that awarded the certificate or license.

Position Summaries

This section of your portfolio should provide descriptions of each position you've held. If possible, include a copy of each position description from the institution. Also include copies of your performance evaluations and examples of articles, projects, or presentations you completed while you were in each position.

Teaching, Research, and Service

Here, highlight your professional development by giving examples of teaching, research, or service activities. Your teaching activities might include descriptions of rotations you precept, student evaluations, course syllabi, lecture outlines, student assignments, and/or printed copies of your presentation slides and other materials. Research activities include thesis work or grant applications, as well as publications or articles you've prepared related to that research. Service activities can involve both volunteer work and your activities with professional societies. Examples of materials that highlight your service work are minutes from meetings where you had a leadership role or flyers from programs you helped organize.

References

Unlike for your résumé and CV, you should include references in your professional portfolio. At a minimum, provide the name, title, and contact information for each reference. Also, consider including detailed descriptions of their relationship to you and a summary of the type of insight they might be able to provide the potential employer.

The Interview

Laurie M. Whalin
2009 PharmD Recipient
Campbell University School of Pharmacy

No matter what strategies and tools you've used to get noticed by a hiring manager—diligent networking, a top-notch résumé—the most critical step in obtaining a job is the interview.

The interview is an opportunity to help employers grasp the benefits they will gain from your skills, experience, and qualifications. They want evidence that you can do the job and that you bring the right interpersonal skills for their needs. Likewise, the interview is your chance to gather the information you need to decide if this is the right position for you. Despite the importance of the interview, many candidates spend more time selecting what to wear than preparing for questions they might be asked.

Preparation is the key to a successful interview. The more you prepare and practice, the more comfortable you'll feel during the interview, which will help you come across as confident and capable. Start getting ready for your interview at least three days to one week before the scheduled appointment.

Do Your Homework

Do as much research as possible about the company or institution where you are interviewing. Learning important facts shows the employer that you are interested in the company and resourceful enough to find relevant information. It also helps you formulate targeted questions to ask during your interview and supplies you with material that might help you answer difficult interview questions.

Box 5-1 lists good sources of information about potential employers and the kinds of information to locate. During your research, take good notes and highlight important facts to memorize in advance.

Being well informed makes you a more desirable candidate and can set you apart from other interviewees. For example, during one of my interviews for a residency, I brought up points I'd read about the institution in a bulletin published by the American Society of Health-System Pharmacists. Afterward, I was told that doing so really impressed the interviewers.

Box 5-1

Where to Find Company Information

Some sources of information about companies where you will be interviewing include:
— Company website
— Company brochures and annual reports
— Articles in magazines or professional journals, which you can find via database searches (accessible via community and university libraries and their websites)
— Business information websites, such as Hoover's (www.hoovers.com)
— Contacts within the profession

Information to identify:
— Location
— Organization structure
— Demographics
— Patient population
— Health care specialties
— Strategic plan
— Mission and vision statements
— Plans to expand services or departments
— Recent company news

Practice Makes Perfect

Begin preparing for your interviews by thoroughly reviewing your résumé or curriculum vitae so you can talk comfortably about your education, experiences, skills, and abilities. Remember, CVs and résumés often serve as prompts for interviewer's questions, so anything they contain is fair game. If your CV lists a presentation you gave during your first year of pharmacy school, for example, you should be able to provide specifics.

When getting ready for my residency interviews, I rehearsed a short summary for each project, presentation, or paper on my CV so I could confidently convey the main points of each in one to two minutes. Then, when interviewers asked me specific questions, I could easily recall the information.

Next, practice answering commonly asked interview questions so you sound poised and professional during the actual interview. Box 5-2 lists some examples of questions, and you can find many more in books about job searching and interviewing. You can also look online by entering search phrases such as "common interview questions" or "job interview questions." Box 5-3 provides a few sources of information on interviews and interview questions.

Advance preparation is especially helpful during behavioral-based interviews, when interviewers ask for specific examples of events in your career and the role you played. (See Interview Formats, page 76, for more information on behavioral interviews). Remembering an event that occurred three years ago can be difficult when you're face-to-face with a potential employer, are feeling nervous, and have limited time.

Creating a list of key projects, activities, and accomplishments and rehearsing points you want to highlight helps you call to mind the most appropriate scenario for each question asked. Also, ask a preceptor or mentor to conduct "mock interviews" with you so you can practice your delivery style, get feedback, and correct flaws or nervous habits before the actual interview.

Box 5-2

Preparing for Interviewers' Questions

It's best to be prepared for a wide range of interview questions, because you never know what you'll be asked or how skilled the interviewer is. Typically, questions probe your background, goals, communication and problem-solving skills, and personal style.

Overall, the question behind everything the interviewer asks you is, "How is this person going to solve my problems or enhance my workplace?" Taking time in advance to think through answers allows you to phrase them in a positive way, highlight accomplishments, and appear poised and confident.

continued on page 70

Box 5-2

continued

Strategies to Get Started

— Be ready to answer the question "Tell me about yourself," which is commonly asked and tough to answer well if you haven't prepared. In your response, spend about a minute on brief details of your education and experience, tying your achievements to the potential employer's needs. Do not include irrelevant information or recount your history from birth. The interviewer is busy and wants a concise, meaningful story.

— Put yourself in the employer's shoes. Think what you would ask if you were the person hiring for this position. Write down at least 10 questions, and then outline answers for each. Do not map out verbatim responses; simply jot the key points you'd want to make.

— Think about interview questions you would find hardest to answer. Write down a few you are most concerned about and, as in the bullet above, outline answers for each.

Sample Questions

1. Tell me how your background qualifies you for this position.
2. Why are you interested in working for this company?
3. What would be your ideal career position?
4. What are your strengths and weaknesses?
5. How would you describe your leadership style?
6. Describe a situation in which you had to request help or assistance on a project.
7. Give an example in which others you were working with on a project disagreed with your ideas. What did you do?
8. Tell me about a time when you failed to meet your own expectations. What did you learn from this?
9. Explain how you stay organized when you have many different projects going at one time.
10. Tell me about a time when you had to deal with a difficult coworker. How did you handle it?
11. Think about a complex project you were assigned. Specifically, what steps did you take to prepare for and finish the project? What was your specific role?
12. Talk about a time when you had to adjust quickly to changes over which you had no control. How did you handle it? How did it impact you directly?
13. Describe a situation in which you had to be assertive to get what you wanted.
14. Give an example of a time when you set a goal and were able to meet or achieve it. Now talk about a time when you set a goal and failed to meet it.
15. Tell me about a time when you had to go above and beyond to get the job done.

Box 5-3

Further Information on Interviewing

The Pharmacy Professional's Guide to Résumés, CVs, & Interviewing
(Reinders TP. 2nd ed. Washington, D.C.: American Pharmacists Association; 2006.)
As its name suggests, this comprehensive text offers advice on everything from
CV and résumé writing to successful interviewing and beyond. It provides sample
interview questions as well as potential questions often asked by interviewers.
As one of the few pharmacy-specific texts in this subject area, this book is my go-to
resource for CV preparation and interviewing. Sample letters for different situations,
such as cover letters, thank-you letters, letters for declining a job offer, and letters
requesting more information make this text an irreplaceable resource on my professional bookshelf.

APhA Career Development Tools
Go to the American Pharmacists Association website at www.pharmacist.com.
Under "APhA Career Development Tools," you'll find links for "Successful Job Inter-
views" and for "Typical Interview Questions" as well as many other helpful resources.

ASHP's CareerPharm
From the American Society of Health-System Pharmacists CareerPharm home page at
www.careerpharm.com, you can find tips for honing your interviewing skills in addition
to information about writing CVs, résumés, cover letters, and thank-you correspondence. Specialized information on "Finding a Job in a Down Market," "Getting Dressed
for the Interview," and "Behavioral Interviews" is also available under the "Interviewing
Skills" drop-down menu.

Tools on ACCP.com
Go to the American College of Clinical Pharmacy home page at www.accp.com and
select "Students" from the menu across the top of the screen. Under the "Career
Development Resources" and "Clinical Compass" tabs you'll find interview tips,
sample questions, and a mock interview video available for download.

Tools on About.com
Go to the home page at www.about.com and select "Job Searching" from the drop-
down menu of topics. Under the "Interviews and Employment" tab you'll find interview
tips and sample questions.

Ask the Right Questions

Usually at some point during an interview, you'll be asked if you have any questions. Your answer should be "yes," and you should be prepared with relevant, insightful questions. Interviewers often rate candidates not just on answers, but on the quality of questions the candidate asks.

Even better than waiting for an invitation is to look for opportunities to ask questions throughout the interview, which shows preparation and initiative and creates two-way communication.

Develop a list of questions to help you understand how your qualifications match the job requirements, evaluate the position and institution, and assess whether this opportunity is a good fit for you.

Pose in-depth questions that can't be answered from the institution's websites or brochures. If you're in the midst of your final residency interview, for example, asking how many staffing hours are required each month isn't a good use of time because you should have obtained that information during your earlier research. Instead you might ask about the types of activities you'd be involved in during a typical shift or what the employer expects you to accomplish during your first six months—beyond what's listed on the job description. Box 5-4 provides sample questions to ask during an interview.

Although I told you to answer "yes" when asked if you have questions—the same advice my mentors gave me—the interview must end at some point. During my residency interviews—typically an all-day process—I made sure I had plenty of useful questions to ask the administrators, preceptors, staff pharmacists, and residents I met. And a time always came when all my questions, and then some, had been answered.

Use your judgment. If you've asked good questions during the interview and feel you've received all the information you need to make a decision about the position, it's okay to say so when the interviewer asks if you have further questions. Express your thanks for the interview. Confirm your interest in the position and briefly summarize your value to the organization. You can also check whether you overlooked any important ways to sell yourself by asking, "What thoughts do you have about my candidacy for this position?"

If you're not sure what the next step will be, ask, "What happens next in your hiring process?" or "When can I expect to hear from you again?"

Box 5-4

Sample Questions to Ask During the Interview

These questions are provided to jumpstart your thinking, but not all are appropriate to ask in every situation. Be sure to develop questions tailored to the position and institution—questions that can't be answered from a brochure or website.

1. What are your institution's strengths and weaknesses?
2. What is the organization's plan for the next five years, and what will be this department's role in that plan?
3. Could you describe your management style? What type of employee do you think will fit in well with that style?
4. What skills and abilities do you feel are necessary for someone to succeed in this position?
5. How will my performance be reviewed, by whom, and how often?
6. Could you describe your ideal employee?
7. How would you describe a typical day/week in this position?
8. Please provide some examples of achievements by others who have held this position.
9. What are some objectives you would like to see accomplished in this job?
10. What significant changes do you see in the near future?
11. What is the biggest challenge I might face if I took this position?
12. What personal qualities or attributes do you value most in your employees, and why?
13. How does the company support professional growth?
14. How would you describe the culture of the organization?
15. Why is this position open?

Logistical Preparation

Nothing makes a worse impression than being late to an interview, no matter what the circumstances. To ensure that this does not happen to you, plan in advance where you are going, how you are going to get there, and what time you need to arrive. Bring with you detailed directions, including information about parking or public transportation if needed.

Arrange to arrive at least 15 to 20 minutes early so you have adequate time to collect yourself and mentally prepare for the day's activities. Make sure you have a clear idea of where you're headed once you arrive at the facility. It's unlikely you'll walk through the front door and find your interviewers waiting to greet you. Probably you'll navigate through several buildings or floors before locating your interview spot. If possible, bring with you a copy of the site map, which can often be found online.

Carry your cell phone and your interviewer's contact information so you can reach him or her if something unexpected prevents you from arriving on time, or you need further directions. Bring cash for such expenses as parking or lunch. Box 5-5 lists items you should have on hand during the interview.

Find out in advance how long the interview is expected to take so you allocate enough time and don't need to worry about missing a bus or your parking meter expiring.

Box 5-5

What to Bring to the Interview

Many institutions will give you an interview itinerary listing materials you need to bring, such as extra copies of your CV or résumé. In case no such list is provided, here are a few staples that should get you through any interview.

- **A small briefcase or professional bag.** Inside, put the few essential belongings you need to carry, such as cell phone (turned off during the interview), business cards, and wallet.
- **Copies of your CV or résumé.** Although most interviewers should already have a copy, it's good to bring 5 to 10 extras you can hand out as needed.
- **List of references with contact information.** Even if you've submitted reference letters prior to the interview, bringing a list of references shows that you are organized, well prepared, and confident in your abilities.
- **Notepad or portfolio with pen or pencil.** Write down notes, comments, or impressions that might be useful to you after the interview as well as reminders about follow-up documents or information you are asked for. Taking notes also demonstrates that you are highly interested and ready to capture important details.
- **Professional portfolio.** Bring your professional portfolio, even if work samples were not requested, to showcase tangible examples of the work you're capable of producing.
- **List of questions for the interviewers.** Bringing the questions you prepared in advance allows you to review them between interview sessions and make note of those you already asked.
- **Copy of interview itinerary, if provided.** You need to know where you are going and who you are interviewing with next, and you can't be sure a duplicate will be available onsite. Not bringing a copy will make you look unprepared and unprofessional.
- **Description of job, residency, or fellowship.** Always bring a copy of the position description, especially if it was provided directly from the institution. This shows that you are prepared, have done your homework, and are ready to seriously discuss your candidacy.

Make a Great Impression

Arrive to the interview looking clean, fresh, and professional. Both men and women should wear neatly pressed, dark, conservative suits with dress shoes. Skirt suits are acceptable for women, but make sure the skirt is long enough to be considered conservative and your legs are covered with pantyhose or tights.

Don't be afraid to inject some personality into your ensemble—just keep it simple. For example, if you decide to wear a brightly colored shirt with detailing under your suit, do not also wear a large, colorful brooch. Use common sense. You want to be remembered for your poise and professionalism—not as the lady or man with the "weird outfit."

It helps to learn a little about the dress code or work environment at the institution where you'll be interviewing. Dress a bit more formally than these guidelines indicate. When it comes to interviews, it is better to err on the side of over-dressed rather than too casual.

Avoid powerful perfumes, colognes, and aftershaves on the day of the interview because strong fragrances can bother interviewers who have allergies or sensitive noses. Make sure your nails are clean and trimmed short. Women wearing nail polish should choose conservative or neutral shades. It's irksome to chip brightly colored polish right before an interview begins—and you have better things to focus on than wondering how you can quickly touch it up.

Cover tattoos and remove any piercings that might be viewed as unprofessional. Earrings are acceptable, but tongue rings or exposed tattoos can leave a poor first impression on a potential employer. As these forms of self-expression become more commonplace, one additional ear piercing for women or an ear piercing for men may be acceptable in some locations. However, you don't want to jeopardize your future career or a great job opportunity over an earring. When in doubt, take it out.

Do not chew gum or smoke during any portion of the interview. Refrain from smoking anywhere on the premises, even on breaks. You never know who you might encounter throughout the day, and you need to make a great impression at all times. Even smoking in your car on the way to the interview can leave a telltale odor on your clothing. If you normally chew gum, try using mints before the interview begins and after any meals.

Greet each interviewer with a firm handshake. Make eye contact and smile—something nervous interviewees often forget. You want to start the interview on the most positive note possible.

Keep nervous habits under control. Without even knowing it, many of us twirl our hair, tap our feet, or fidget with our hands when we're nervous. Be aware of and limit these distracting, unprofessional behaviors. Sit with your hands folded in your lap and lean in slightly so you appear to be actively participating in the conversation.

Also, stay away from filler words such as "um," "you know," and "like" while you think about what to say next. When you're asked a difficult question, it's perfectly acceptable to say, "That was a great question—let me think about it for a moment." Answer confidently and completely when you're ready, and avoid those annoying filler words.   A few other things to remember:

— **Don't mention what you can't do.** Even if you're asked directly about a specific skill or experience, never say you can't do something. Instead talk about an experience that relates to the skill, so the interviewer knows you will at least be capable of learning.

— **Don't lie.** When elaborating on certain experiences, always be truthful. Lies have a tendency to surface again, and pharmacy is a small world. If you don't know something, admit it rather than trying to wing it. No one can be knowledgeable about everything.

— **Never speak negatively about past jobs, supervisors, or coworkers.** If you're asked directly about your least favorite rotation or preceptor, focus on the tasks or learning styles you like best compared to others. Never get personal.

— **Don't bring up topics such as salary, benefits, or bonuses during the interview.** Wait until after you have received an offer. Use your interview time to talk about skills and attributes you can bring to the company.

— **Ask questions.** The interview is your chance to find out if the company is a good match for you.

— **Focus on your accomplishments.** This is your time to shine! Many people feel silly or egotistical talking about themselves. But you have a limited time to sell yourself for the position, so don't hold back.

Interview Formats

Interviews can be conducted in many ways. The format typically depends on the institution itself and the position for which you are interviewing.

One-on-One Interviews

One of the most common interview formats is when one person interviews a candidate individually. Sometimes an additional staff member, such as an assistant director or manager, might be present to help in the interview process.

Panel Interviews

In this scenario, several interviewers—usually from different departments or specialties—interview the candidate at one time. This format is typical in both educational and governmental settings. One interviewer might take the lead, with other members of the panel interjecting occasionally, or you might face a barrage of questions from all members of the panel.

Serial Interviews

In this approach, commonly used for residencies or fellowships, you meet with several different interviewers or groups of interviewers back to back. During these types of interviews, it's important to treat each interview as if it's your first, even if you're asked questions you already answered, and to be consistent in your replies. When interviewers compare notes later, you want them to have formulated the same impression.

Group Interviews

Group interviews gather several interviewers and candidates together in one session. These types of interviews highlight your interpersonal and leadership skills, as well as your ability to handle stressful situations. Interviewers will be assessing the behaviors you display in the group setting, so it is important to maintain balanced interactions and avoid being overly aggressive.

Phone Interviews

Employers may use phone interviews as a more cost-effective method of screening applicants before offering on-site interviews to selected candidates. Phone interviews may also be used when schedules or geography prevent meeting in person. Most of the tips for other kinds of interviews are also applicable to those conducted by telephone. Speak slowly and enunciate. Limit your responses to concise, clear answers. Keep at hand a copy of any materials you sent when applying for the position, such as your CV, résumé, or letter of intent, because interviewers may reference these items during the call.

Set aside enough time for the interview and plan to take the call in a quiet, distraction-free location—someplace where dogs won't bark and no music wafts in the background. Landlines tend to have better clarity, but if you must use your cell phone, be sure it's well charged, you have a good signal, and you're planted in a quiet room—not driving or walking.

Know ahead of time whom you'll be speaking with and who will call whom. If the employer will be calling you, clearly designate the phone number they should use to reach you on the scheduled date and time. If it's up to you to call, be prompt. Some interviewers use a conference call system with a dial-in number and access code; have all phone-in details handy so you're not scrambling at the last minute. If multiple parties will be on the call, get their full names, titles, and the proper spelling in advance, because it's hard to discern names and voices on a conference call.

As with other types of interviews, have prepared questions ready and send correspondence thanking the interviewers for their time once the call is complete.

Types of Interviews

Interviews might involve specific techniques and types of questions, depending on their purpose.

Traditional Interviews

Traditional interviews typically focus on your management or leadership style, your attributes and beliefs, and how you would handle hypothetical situations. Strictly traditional interviews have become less favored among interviewers, but traditional interview questions are often mixed in with behavioral-type questions.

Examples of traditional interview questions include "Tell me about yourself" and "Where would you like to be in five years?" When answering traditional questions, first state what you know how to do, then give an example of that skill, knowledge, or characteristic, and last, explain the benefit that skill will bring to the organization.

Answer most questions within 60 seconds. If the interviewer would like you to elaborate, he or she can ask a follow-up question.

Behavioral Interviews

Behavioral interviews, based on the premise that past behaviors are the best predictors of future performance, are becoming increasingly popular. Unlike traditional interviews in which candidates can often give "canned" answers conveying what they think interviewers want to hear, behavioral interviews are designed to elicit specific descriptions of past actions.

Examples of behavioral interview questions include, "Describe a situation in which you motivated yourself to complete a task or assignment you did not want to do," or "Give me an example of a time when you had to make a split-second decision."

To answer behavioral-based questions, keep in mind the mnemonic device "STAR."
- **Situation:** Describe a specific situation that addresses the question.
- **Task:** Explain the task associated with the situation.
- **Action:** List the actions you took to address the situation.
- **Result:** Describe the results you obtained and how they benefited your employer or organization.

Answers to behavioral-based questions are significantly longer than those for traditional interview questions, with the average answer lasting around three minutes.

Case-Based Interviews

For at least part of your interview, you might be asked to complete a case study, perform a task, or undergo an examination. Typically, you will be presented with a patient case and then will be asked a series of questions regarding the patient's disease states and potential therapies. Tips for answering case-based interview questions include:
- Read *all* the information provided and follow directions carefully. The case might contain explicit instructions you need to follow, such as page limits.
- Make appropriate use of your time. You might want to make an outline of things to include in your case study. Be sure to leave yourself enough time to answer all the questions, however.
- Clearly state any assumptions you are making about your patient or the patient's therapy, so the interviewer knows exactly what you are thinking.
- Answer all questions. Although the purpose of the case is to evaluate your critical thinking skills, you need to respond to each question to the best of your ability.

Stress Interviews

This uncommon type of interview is designed to see how well you handle pressure as well as when and how you assert yourself. Interviewers might try to rattle you by acting rude or sarcastic, disagreeing, remaining silent for long periods, or asking several questions in a row before allowing you to answer. The key to surviving stress interviews is to remain calm and avoid taking the actions personally.

During the Interview

The best advice I've heard for enhancing your performance during an interview is to speak in specifics and translate your interests, skills, and values into something concrete.

For example, if you say "I work well with people" or "I'm a hard worker," you're mentioning good traits but you're not telling interviewers what they need to know—how you can contribute to the organization.

Instead try to say something like, "Our school was told by the accreditation committee that we needed to start a tutoring program specifically for the school of pharmacy. As president of the pharmaceutical honor society at my school, I was in charge of organizing this process. I developed the student referral plan for tutoring, handled all administrative duties, including developing referral forms and scheduling, and trained honor society members to be tutors. The tutoring program was up and running within the semester, is still in place, and continues to help pharmacy students at my university today."

The type of response above allows interviewers to recognize through your actions that you're a hard worker, rather than taking your word for it, and helps them visualize the role you'll play and benefits you'll bring to their organization.

After the Interview

Evaluate your performance after each interview, identifying your strengths and weaknesses and making note of things to do differently next time. Each interview is a learning experience, helping you enhance your interviewing skills and avoid repeating the same mistakes. Questions to ask yourself include:
- Did I highlight my experience and skills to show the interviewer what I offer to the job?
- Did I talk too much or too little?
- Did I ask questions that helped me clarify the job and showed my interest?

Following each interview, list your feelings regarding staff interactions, work environment, and opportunities for advancement. Do this right away, while your thoughts are fresh. You need to evaluate whether the position is in line with your expectations and goals, both immediate and long term. Ask yourself, "Can I see myself working here every day?" and "Can I see myself working with this group of people?" Then when you need to make a decision about the position, you can refer back to clear written impressions rather than relying on cloudy memories.

Always send a thank-you letter regardless of your interest in the position or how well you think the interview went. Within a day or two after the interview date, send a thank-you letter to your primary contact at the organization. Also consider sending notes to everyone you met during the day of the interview, especially those with whom you spent a significant amount of time.

Your thank-you letter reminds interviewers of who you are and can make you stand out in a sea of applicants. Thank-you letters should express thanks for the interviewers' time and effort, reaffirm your interest in the position, and emphasize a few of your principal skills. Remember to include your contact information for follow-up, and state that you are always available to answer additional questions that the selection committee might have before making a decision. Figures 5-1 and 5-2 on pages 83 and 84 give examples of well-crafted thank-you letters.

Eventually, you'll find yourself in the position of interviewer. Box 5-6 provides tips for conducting yourself productively when that day comes.

Box 5-6

When You're the Interviewer
by Jennifer P. Askew

At some point in your career, you'll be the one doing the interviewing—as happened to me when I was barely out of pharmacy school. I was in a residency program and was asked to help interview potential candidates for the following year. I picked them up from their hotel, transported them to the hospital, accompanied them on their lunch outing, and later shared my impressions to help select the best candidates.

Your first experience with the interview process might be informal, like mine, or you might be part of a formal interview team. Either way, you can start preparing now by noticing the tactics that work well when you're going through interviews. Observation is a great way to learn. Here are a few tips to keep in mind.

- **Don't be nosy.** Avoid the temptation to ask personal questions about candidates or their background, which is not only intrusive but in some cases—such as age, religion, or marital status—is illegal.
- **Don't ask yes-no questions.** Asking open-ended questions that can't be answered with "yes" or "no" helps you get to know the candidate and obtain deeper information. In fact, yes-no questions can be leading, such as, "You know how to counsel a patient on the proper use of an inhaler, right?"
- **Don't talk too much.** If candidates receive an appropriate amount of background information in advance, you don't have to spend your time providing it during the interview. Use the time to get to know the candidate.
- **Don't compare candidates to each other.** Employ the same set of criteria to evaluate each applicant on his or her own merits rather than using another candidate as a yardstick.
- **Do your homework.** Read the applicant's cover letter and CV or résumé to get an idea of his or her background. Don't waste interview time asking things you could have learned from preparing properly.

continued on page 82

Box 5-6

continued

- **Talk about expectations and goals.** Make sure the applicant knows what is going to be expected of someone who fills the role for which you are interviewing.
- **Ask behavior-based questions.** As mentioned earlier in this chapter, such questions give you specific examples of a candidate's skills or traits in action, including the results. If you don't get the whole story, ask probing questions, such as "And then what happened?"or "Can you be more specific?"
- **Write it down.** You might think you'll be able to remember every detail when it's time to evaluate the applicant, but you won't, especially if you're interviewing multiple candidates over an extended period of time. Jot down key concepts, responses, or qualities to jog your memory when the time comes.

Figure 5-1

Sample Thank-You Letter for Residency Interview

Abigail D. Martin
2865 North Fourth Street, Kilmarnock, VA 89635
(865) 894-8246   amartin@email.unc.edu

May 6, 2010

Ezekiel Z. Ellsworth, PharmD
Director of Pharmacy Services
Savannah Regional Hospital
541 Spanish Moss Drive
Savannah, GA 83256

Re: Resident Match Number 39715

Dear Dr. Ellsworth:

Thank you so much for inviting me to interview for your pharmacy practice residency program. I appreciate the time that you and your staff devoted to me during the interview session.

I am very interested in completing a pharmacy practice residency under your guidance. After going through the on-site interview process, I am even more convinced that your program is a great fit for me. I particularly enjoyed learning more about the variety of electives offered at your site, as well as the new pediatric rotation, among other strengths. My motivation and strong work ethic will allow me to contribute a great deal to your institution if I am selected for your program.

Please let me know if your staff needs any additional information before you conclude the residency match process. You are welcome to reach me via email or phone anytime.

Sincerely,

Abigail D. Martin

Figure 5-2

Sample Thank-You Letter for Job Interview

Luke M. O'Bryan, PharmD

3962 Slomba Drive
Asheville, NC 34961
(862) 739-1526
lmobryan@yahoo.com

March 14, 2010

Henry R. Sanford, PharmD
Family Community Pharmacy
5264 Rothstein Drive
San Diego, CA 56798

Dear Dr. Sanford:

Thank you for the opportunity to interview with you and your staff. I appreciate the time and effort you spent in organizing this informative session.

I am very interested in joining your community pharmacy staff and contributing my skills to your high-quality operation. I am particularly impressed by your emphasis on clinical pharmacy services and local health screenings.

My community pharmacy residency training has prepared me to provide significant contributions to Family Community Pharmacy. I have experience providing one-on-one counseling about diabetes, hypertension, and smoking cessation and am trained to administer immunizations. I'm known for my positive outlook, upbeat demeanor with patients, listening skills, and ability to deliver clear, concise information.

Please let me know if you need additional information about my qualifications or experience. I look forward to hearing from you soon.

Sincerely,

Luke M. O'Bryan, PharmD

Handling the Job Offer

How exciting to receive a job offer! And how overwhelming to weigh all the factors involved and make a decision. Your decision-making challenges are compounded if you receive several offers. How should you proceed?

First, get each offer in writing—either by email, fax, or standard mail delivery. If your offer comes in by phone and there's no mention of written information on the way, ask for it. It's hard to assess the offer without reading it in black and white.

Also ask for a copy of the proposed job description, if you don't have it already, to make sure you and your potential employer are on the same page about how your activities will be prioritized. Some employers will send you a package of background information on benefits, the local community, and other topics that may help as you consider the offer. If the company doesn't tell you this package is coming, go ahead and request the information you need.

When the offer arrives, it's fine to ask if you can discuss the job specifics in person or by phone. Simply request an appointment to talk; don't assume that the person has time to speak with you on the spot. Be specific about whom you want to talk with—your future supervisor, a human resources representative, or both, for example—and ask to schedule time at their convenience, to avoid seeming rude or inconsiderate.

You must consider many things when choosing a job, and when it's your first professional position, it can feel as if your entire future rides on making the right decision. Some choices may be better for you than others, but it's rare for a decision to be flat-out wrong.

Even so, I recommend that you avoid accepting the first job offer that comes your way—no matter how anxious you are to get past the search and into the workplace. Hold out for a position that feels like a good fit.

Think of your advantages. You've recently completed training, which means you are prepared with the most up-to-date information in the field. Also, you can evaluate several different jobs simultaneously, unlike pharmacists out in practice who are searching for a new position while holding down full-time work.

Many opportunities will come your way. Relax—and use both your head and your heart to decide.

Using a Rubric

Some simple techniques can help objectify your decision—along with the same common sense you've used when making other difficult personal and professional decisions. For example, the scoring rubric used in Chapter 3 to help you choose a career path can easily be adapted for your job decision, as shown in Figure 6-1.

Simply insert criteria that reflect concrete factors such as retirement plans, vacation time, allowance for professional time and expenses, and insurance for disability, life, and health. Figure 6-1 gives some suggested categories to include, but you can adjust them any way that works for you.

Chances are, when you receive an offer, you won't yet have all the information you need to complete the rubric and make a decision. Job interviews are not the time to ask for details on salary and benefits. But once you've been given an offer, you must gather the specifics.

Benefits

The benefits and perks you receive through your employment are an important part of your compensation. In fact, employment benefits can make up 40% or more of your total package.

Typically employers have a benefits handbook that explains the full scope of benefits and details about each. Ask to review a copy. Then follow up to get information that the handbook doesn't cover in sufficient detail. Below is a list of information you should obtain for each benefit.

– How much the benefit will cost you, if anything. Does the employer pay all or some of the cost? What portion must you pay yourself?

Figure 6-1

Rubric for Evaluating Job Offers

Directions: Determine the level of importance of each criterion and assign a weighting factor based on how much it matters to you. This importance is expressed as a percentage of the total, just as it was in the example in Chapter 3. Your weighting factors should total 100%. Remember you can have as many or as few criteria as you like. You can also combine criteria into categories as in the example below. Once your list of criteria is weighted, use the rating scale below to assign a rating for each criterion pertaining to each position.

Rating Scale: Unacceptable (1) to Ideal (10)

Criteria	Weighting Factor (%)	Position A		Position B		Position C	
		Rating (1-10)	Total Score (Weight x Rating)	Rating (1-10)	Total Score (Weight x Rating)	Rating (1-10)	Total Score (Weight x Rating)
Position (Match to your knowledge, skills, and attitudes)	30%	6	1.8	7	2.1	4	1.2
Organization (Size, management structure, reputation, opportunities for advancement, work environment)	30%	8	2.4	9	2.7	8	2.4
Geographic Location (Cost of living, housing availability, climate)	10%	3	0.3	6	0.6	5	0.5
Lifestyle Issues (Schedule, commute time, social activities)	15%	5	0.8	4	0.6	7	1.1
Compensation (Salary and benefits)	15%	5	0.8	8	1.2	9	1.4
Total	**100%**		**6.1**		**7.2**		**6.6**

- When and how the benefit is paid for. For example, is it taken out of your regular paycheck, pre-tax?
- Who is eligible. Some benefits may be offered only to you, and others may be extended to your spouse or children.
- The process for enrolling in each benefit, including whether you enroll upfront, anytime, or at a designated time during the year.
- When you are eligible—immediately? After a certain amount of time on the job?
- Will you be taxed on the benefit?

Medical Plans

You will want to know what type of health care plan is offered. Specific information to obtain includes:
- The expenses that are covered.
- The cost of copayments and deductibles.
- Exclusion criteria for pre-existing conditions.
- Enrollment criteria, such as a required medical exam.

Some of the most popular types of health care plans are:
- **Health Maintenance Organization (HMO).** Typically you choose a primary care physician from a list of providers in the network. Any supplemental care by specialists, such as dermatologists or cardiologists, is provided by referral from this primary care provider you have chosen. Care is typically prepaid with a fixed monthly fee, regardless of the amount of care needed, in HMO plans. An HMO may cost less than other plans, but also provides less flexibility.
- **Preferred Provider Organization (PPO).** These groups of physicians, hospitals, and other providers are similar in some ways to HMOs, but you can usually see any physician or specialist and go to any hospital or medical practice. You typically pay more, however, to see providers or use facilities that are not on the PPO list of preferred providers. With most PPO plans, you pay for care (or at least pay your predetermined copay) at the time it is rendered.
- **Point of Service (POS) Plan.** Falling somewhere between HMOs and PPOs in terms of the cost of care and choices offered, POS plans typically cover services in an HMO-style model with care directed by a primary care physician. You can also choose to seek care outside the POS network, at added expense to you, similar to a PPO.

Your employer may offer separate plans for the following:
- **Dental**. You will want to know whether preventive care, orthodontics, and surgical needs are covered and to what extent.
- **Vision/Eye**. Even if you don't need it now, most people will require ophthalmologic services at some point during their lifetime. Find out which services are covered and to what extent. Many plans offer an annual "allowance" that can cover eye exams, corrective lenses, and other needs.

Other Benefits and Insurance

Other types of benefits and coverage your employer is likely to offer are listed below, along with information you should obtain for each.

Life Insurance

If you're young, this benefit might not seem terribly important to you, but as you grow older and raise a family, you'll see it differently because it helps provide for your family if something happens to you. Find out how much coverage is offered and what the options are for purchasing additional blocks of coverage. If you can't buy additional coverage at work, keep in mind that you can usually buy it from insurance companies without going through your employer.

Short- and Long-Term Disability

This type of insurance covers what the names suggest—allowing you to receive income if you are unable to work because of sickness or injury. Short-term disability covers a briefer time, usually up to about six months, while long-term disability covers a more extended period. You will want to know the percentage of your salary you will receive if you become disabled and how the percentage may change over time.

Think you don't need it? Studies show that a 20-year-old worker has a 30% chance of becoming disabled before reaching retirement age, according to the Social Security Administration.

401(k) Retirement Savings Plan

In this type of retirement plan, your employer deposits a portion of your wages directly into your 401(k) account to help you save. The tax-deferred savings are invested—usually according to a mix of investments you select from a portfolio of options. Many employers also deposit an additional amount or "match" into your account, which is based on how much you contribute and is capped by a predetermined limit. Retirement may not seem that important now, but the earlier you start investing, the more money you will have when you're ready to stop working.

Pension

Traditional pension plans are, for the most part, being replaced by 401(k) plans. In a typical pension plan, your company puts a predetermined amount of money into an account for you that silently accumulates over time.

Paid Time Off

This benefit category includes vacation, personal days, sick days, and holidays. Some employers have separate sets of rules for each type of time off, and some consider all days off, no matter what the reason, to be "paid time off" or PTO. In some situations, the potential employer's benefits department will designate how and when you are

allowed time off; in other cases, that duty is delegated to your supervisor—which means you might need to inquire about PTO with both. Find out:
- How many days you are allowed off.
- What type of notice is required to take these days off—a written request? How many days in advance?
- Which days the employer considers holidays.
- How many holidays you will likely have to work.
- When your PTO starts accumulating and how much you receive per pay period.
- Whether your PTO must be earned before it is used, or whether PTO can be advanced to you before you have earned it.
- If any unused PTO can be rolled over to subsequent years and what the rules are.
- Whether you can "sell back" any unused PTO.

Professional Time and Expense Allowance

Some employers offer you paid time away from the office that does not count as vacation or personal time if you spend it on activities that benefit the employer or make you a better or more knowledgeable employee. The employer may also cover some of your expenses related to professional activities.

For example, if you're attending the American Pharmacists Association Annual Meeting to present a poster about a project you're working on, your employer may allow you one or more days off work without counting it as vacation and may even help with part of your registration fee or travel expenses. Be sure to find out the employer's policy for such events, including how much time off and which expenses will be covered.

Other Expense Reimbursement

Depending on where you live and work, some employers might also provide reim-bursement for commuting costs, parking fees, or other business-related costs. Learn which expenses will be covered and to what extent.

Dependent Care

Some employers have an on-site facility for child care. Some might provide an allow-ance to spend on child care or have the ability to set aside pre-tax dollars from your pay for you to put toward child care or elder care, if needed.

Tuition Reimbursement

If you're just finishing up your pharmacy studies, "school" is probably the last word you want to hear. But if you decide to go back for further education, such as a Mas-ter's in Business Administration (MBA) or a Master's in Public Health (MPH), it's a huge help if your employer pays part of your expenses through a tuition reimbursement program. Some employers will also contribute toward expenses to obtain advanced credentials, such as those obtained through the Board of Pharmacy Specialties. As with the other benefits, you'll want to know what types of education are covered and to what extent.

Liability Insurance

Most employers in the pharmacy field will provide you with liability coverage as long as you are "on the clock" and operating within the scope of your practice and job description—but you'll want to verify that this is the case. If your employer does not offer liability insurance or you feel that the insurance provided does not cover your activities completely, check out Healthcare Providers Service Organization (HPSO), found at www.hpso.com, to find coverage on your own.

Some pharmacy associations, such as the American Pharmacists Association, offer discounted liability coverage as a benefit of membership. In my case, I choose to keep additional coverage because I do a lot of volunteer and service work outside the scope of my regular, full-time job, and I want to be sure I'm covered in all situations. For the small amount I pay for additional coverage, it is worth the peace of mind.

Health Clubs

Some employers have on-site fitness facilities or make provisions for reduced membership rates at local health clubs. Some pay your fitness club dues entirely. At first glance this may not seem like an important aspect of a future position, but add-on options such as health club membership can really help you save your hard-earned money in the long run. And this benefit tells you that the employer gives more than lip service to preventive health measures and your well-being.

Employee Assistance

Employers might offer many different types of assistance, including financial counseling, tax preparation services, crisis support, and even anonymous alcohol and drug counseling. Such programs might not be on your list of "must-have" benefits, but they could be a useful value-added service, if a potential employer offers them.

Overtime or Comp Time

If you are looking at salaried positions, you are typically ineligible for overtime pay, but the employer may offer bonus or "premium" pay for working nights or holidays or at out-of-town locations. The employer may also offer "comp" time, which allows you to accrue additional time off for extra hours you work.

Medical Expense Accounts

Several options exist for employers to provide accounts you can use to pay for health care expenses not otherwise covered by the employer's health plan. Common names are health savings accounts, flexible spending accounts, and health reimbursement accounts; for each, there can be differences in tax treatment, who can contribute, and what expenses are covered. These accounts allow you to set aside pre-tax dollars to spend on many different types of medical expenses, from fees for doctor's office visits to prescriptions, contact lenses, and certain over-the-counter medications.

Salary

At the top of your mind is no doubt the *big* question. "How much am I going to get paid?" When you're offered a salary, you should be able to evaluate how it compares with averages in your field.

Research Average Salaries

First, you must do a little research. Then you can rank the salaries offered and fill in your rubric in Figure 6-1. You should find out what other people are making who:
- Are in similar positions to the one you are being offered.
- Have a similar amount of work experience as you.
- Work in a similar geographic area.

Although all these considerations are important, one or more may be *more* important depending on where you want to work and the types of jobs you're looking for. For example, if you're considering a staff pharmacist position at the only hospital in a small rural community, that hospital may be competing with other types of employers to hire staff pharmacists, such as community pharmacies and long-term care facilities. So in this example, geography is likely to be a better predictor of your potential salary than other factors and it will be important to find out what pharmacists are being paid in the local area. Looking at salaries for hospital staff pharmacists in other geographic areas, while still important, may be less critical.

On the other hand, if you want to be a community staff pharmacist in a large metropolitan area where many community pharmacies are located, employers may be competing with other community pharmacies for pharmacists with more experience. In this case, the amount of experience a candidate brings to the table probably has a bearing on the salary offered. It would be important to find out what pharmacists are being paid who have background and experience similar to yours.

The most simple, informal way to research salaries is by asking around—tapping the people in your network. If you've recently finished pharmacy school or postgraduate training, you probably have classmates or colleagues who are job hunting, too. Stay connected with them and, very professionally of course, compare notes about salary ranges. Other ways to research salaries include:

- **Pharmacy publications and news magazines.** For example, *Drug Topics* publishes annual survey results about average pharmacist salaries in the U.S. broken down by regions, such as the Southwest or Northeast.
- **Salary finder services.** Several services, for a small fee, will assess the average market and salary for a particular job in a particular geographic area. An example is Salary.com, which offers a "Personal Salary Report."
- **Online sources.** Many recruiting agencies, career-finder websites, and other groups post average salaries online.

Raises

Once you know how much you can expect to make, based on the job title, your experience, and geography, you can determine whether the salary being offered is average, above average, or below average. Also consider the cost of living for the area and additional expenses such as parking or transportation (mass transit, highway tolls).

Don't forget raises when you're evaluating the pay you can expect at a potential employer. Ask if raises are tied to performance reviews and how often these take place. Keep in mind that cost-of-living pay increases are not raises (although you'll want to ask about those, too).

The article "Negotiate a Raise in Healthcare" on Monster.com notes that the health care industry tends to have rigid salary structures, so the best time to negotiate a salary increase is when you're interviewing for the job. Once you're on board, you may be locked into a strict schedule for raises—especially at large companies.

Raises can also take the form of promotions. You may have heard that the pay a pharmacist receives immediately out of school is not much different from the pay later in his or her career. Although that's true in some situations, a growing number of employers are finding ways to reward experience or expertise through promotions, bonuses, raises, and other perks. For example, some hospital pharmacy departments are developing career ladders to improve staff retention. With every rung ascended, the pharmacist gets more responsibilities, such as precepting students or handling advanced clinical practice requirements, and also gets a commensurate increase in pay.

Resources and Relocation

To remind yourself of other items to consider, pull out the notes you took during your interviews. Was a cell phone or mobile device included with the position? How about an office, computer, laptop, printer, or other resources? Are relocation expenses covered? This review helps you think through how the employer you are evaluating stacks up against others you met with.

Box 6-1 lists sources of additional information on factors to consider and how to evaluate job offers.

Box 6-1

Further Reading on Evaluating Job Offers

APhA Career Development Tools
Go to the American Pharmacists Association website at www.pharmacist.com. Under "APhA Career Development Tools" click the link for "Evaluating Job Offers."

Bureau of Labor Statistics
This bureau within the Department of Labor, found at www.bls.gov, publishes useful job search information. On the website, click the "Publications" tab and scroll down to the "Career Guides" section. Click on the *Occupational Outlook Handbook*. The "Job Search Tips" section has helpful information about evaluating a job offer.

Collegegrad.com
The College grad website offers lots of job search advice. Go to www.collegegrad.com/jobsearch and click the "Offer" box in the navigation column. You'll find tips on negotiating and evaluating jobs, as well as a great "Job Offer Checklist."

The 'Heart' Part

In addition to the tangible parts of the employment package, you must assess the less quantifiable aspects. For example:

– How do you feel about your would-be supervisor? Can you see yourself being happy working for this person?
– How about your would-be colleagues? Do they seem like people you could collaborate with and work alongside?
– How does the company's atmosphere feel to you?
– Are the company's interests and values compatible with yours?

Such considerations may seem like uncharted territory, but you've surely done this kind of decision-making before. When I was planning my undergraduate studies, my family and I toured the campuses of three universities that really interested me. At two, I felt at ease. I enjoyed the landscaping and the sight of people reading, studying, and playing Frisbee in grassy areas between buildings. People seemed welcoming; libraries and study areas looked comfortable and inviting.

At the third school, people weren't rude, but they didn't seem as friendly. The campus was beautiful, but I couldn't picture myself there each day. The libraries and study areas seemed a little cold and stiff. I was accepted by all three, and two scored highly on the rubric of criteria I'd established. When deciding between those two, intangibles made all the difference. I felt at ease at one school, and I didn't at the other. My decision was made.

Be sure to add some intangible "heart" criteria to your rubric—and make sure these criteria come from *your* heart. Don't confuse your feelings about a particular job with those of your parents, professors, or mentors.

You may not call them "heart" criteria in your rubric—they are simply factors that matter a lot to you personally. For example, the size of the institution may be important to you. Will you be happiest at a large, prestigious institution or would you rather be a big fish in a small pond? Do you want to be geographically close to an ailing relative? Are you a competitive skier who seeks mountains nearby so you can continue to train? If a job lacks some of your "heart" criteria, it doesn't mean you shouldn't consider it—other positives may outweigh what's missing. Filling out the rubric helps you figure out how jobs stack up against each other.

Buying Time

Evaluating a job offer takes time. How do you tell a future employer that you need to think things over without sounding rude or uninterested? With honesty.

I don't mean it's okay to say, "Thank you for the offer, but you're really my second choice. Once I hear from my first choice, I'll let you know." Be both honest and professional, like this:
— Thank the employer for the offer.
— Ask for the offer in writing, unless the employer has told you it's already on its way.
— Say that you are in the process of interviewing with several potential employers.
— Give a date when you will be back in touch with your decision. This date should be within the next few days, or a couple of weeks at the most. Then be sure to give your answer by the promised date.

For example, you might say, "Thank you so much for the offer. I can't wait to read all the details you are sending via email. Just to keep us on the same page, I have two more interviews coming up, but I should be all done by next Friday. Would it be all right for me to give you a call about my decision then?"

Negotiating and Accepting

If you collected all the information you need about each opportunity and filled out your rubric, making your decision should be relatively easy. Just remember that when you accept the offer, you are agreeing to the salary, benefits, and job description as presented.

Many things can be negotiated, not just salary. For example, if you want to devote a certain amount of time to teaching or precepting, ask for it to be added to your job description. Do you hope to work from home one day a week or designate time for work-related projects? Ask. If there's something you really want or need, get it coming in the door—*before* you accept the positon—because once you're on board, you have very little leverage for negotiating.

For example, let's say you'd like to say yes to a position, but you want to designate one half-day per week to specific projects. Contact the potential employer to request that your job description be amended to reflect this activity. Be diplomatic. You could say something like, "Just to make sure my request doesn't get lost in the shuffle when I come on board, will you please add one half-day of project time per week to my job description?" You can also make your request by email, which helps you get it in writing; the response serves as the confirmation or denial of your request.

Before you make the request, decide whether you're willing to live without the item you are negotiating. That way, you won't be put on the spot. If you're not willing to take the job without the half-day of project time and your future employer will not agree, politely decline the offer and thank the potential employer for his or her time. As long as you are professional, there is nothing wrong with turning down a job offer that does not provide what you're looking for.

If the term "negotiation" has a negative connotation for you, consider that all you're doing is communicating with your potential employer. You are setting expectations and ensuring that needs are met on both sides. There are no hard and fast rules for negotiating about your job offer. Be honest, professional, and open in your communications, and pin down the details in writing.

Accepting

Even if you've accepted a job by phone, it's a good idea to send a brief job acceptance letter to the person who offered you the position. The letter should:
- Thank the employer for the opportunity.
- State that you accept the position.
- Confirm the key terms and conditions of employment, such as salary and benefits.
- Include any items that have been negotiated during your acceptance of the position.
- Confirm your starting date of employment.

An acceptance letter is a professional touch, but also a valuable record, compiling key information in one document you can easily retrieve. Later, when you're seeking other positions, you can quickly look up your start date, starting salary, and other facts that applications may require.

Declining

If you decide a particular offer is not for you, be polite and professional in declining the offer. You never know when you will cross paths with that employer again. You might even want to work there someday in the future. Make sure to leave behind a positive impression. If you haven't learned it already, pharmacy is a *very* small world.

Because voice conveys tone so much better than writing, it's best to decline the offer by telephone rather than sending an email or letter, which can seem cold and distant in such circumstances. Thank the employer for the opportunity and say something specific about the company that impressed you. Without going into a lot of detail, explain that you are taking another position that will allow you to contribute a specific skill or talent that matters to you. Keep the call brief, and come across in a heartfelt and positive way. Then follow up in writing. You can also use a letter or email if you simply can't reach the person by phone who offered the position.

The Pharmacy Professional's Guide to Résumés, CVs, & Interviewing, which is cited in several resource lists in this book, offers a selection of template letters you can use for declining a job offer, in addition to templates for accepting a job.

Adjusting to the Workplace

Adjusting to the work environment can be one of the most stressful aspects of your first job. Everything seems new and different, and you have a whole new set of responsibilities. This chapter addresses some of the most challenging aspects, from what to expect on your first day to how to work well with your boss, and provides strategies to make the transition as smooth as possible. If you'd like to read more about topics covered here, Box 7-1 on page 101 suggests additional resources.

Your Schedule

Your schedule as a practicing pharmacist is likely to be very different from the schedule you maintained as a student. Personally, I went from having plenty of built-in "down time" or "study time" to a much more packed timetable. Not to mention that spring breaks and summer vacations are now things of the past.

Some schedules will call for you to work eight hours a day, five days a week, while others may require four 10-hour days or some other arrangement. Some of you will have to work nights, weekends, or holidays, either regularly or periodically. You may be paid hourly (called "non-exempt" in some companies) or make a salary (exempt). You may even get called something bizarre like "0.8 FTE" or "0.6 FTE," which does not mean that you count as a fraction of a person, but conveys your "full time equivalency." If a typical employee works 40 hours per week, 0.8 FTE means you work only 32 hours.

One of the easiest ways to adjust to a new schedule is to set up a routine for yourself. Here are some suggestions.

Step 1: Calendar

Start with an empty calendar. I prefer to use my Pocket PC, because it connects with my computer and allows me to access or update my calendar quickly and easily. You may choose a daily planner or even a simple electronic spreadsheet, if you prefer. There are also calendars on most personal email systems, such as Hotmail and Yahoo!

Step 2: Work Schedule

First, "pencil in" your work time. Do you have to be at work the same time every day? Some days, are you required to come in early or stay late? Do you have the same schedule every week or every month? Or does your schedule change? Map out a few months to see how it looks once it's written down.

Step 3: Daily, Weekly, and Monthly Routine

Now, take a moment to list the things you need to do daily, weekly, or monthly. How many days do you exercise each week? Put that on the list. Do you have a regular date night, guys' night, or girls' night out? Put that on the list. How many times per week do you usually need to grocery shop or run other errands? Put that on the list, too.

Then start plugging the items into your calendar. Does going to the gym fit in best before or after work? Would going to the grocery store work better on a weeknight or on the weekend? There's no need to follow this schedule religiously, but having some idea of how things fit in will prevent you from reaching the end of a week or month and finding you've left out something you meant to do.

For example, I got really busy during one period early in my career and failed to make exercise a priority. I wasn't training for a marathon—but I needed the minimum 20 to 30 minutes of cardiovascular exercise three to five times a week, and I wasn't getting it. I discovered it was much harder to shed the extra 30 pounds and get fit enough to play sports than it would have been to stay in shape in the first place. This experience motivated me to take better charge of my calendar.

You should even plan for something we take for granted—sleep. The average person needs eight hours per night. How much do you require? Approximately what time, in your new work schedule, should you go to sleep and wake up? Avoid the trap of telling yourself you can make do with less sleep than you actually need, like I did. I'd think, "most people need eight, but I'm fine with six," when I should have been thinking, "most people need eight, but that's not enough to leave me rested and refreshed." I was kidding myself! I love sleep! And I need a lot of it to function properly. That doesn't mean I'm not a hard worker or that I'll be less successful than someone who skimps on sleep. But I learned to listen to my body, understand my needs, and accommodate them in a positive way. On days when I have a big project to finish, maybe I can't sleep as much as I'd like or get to the gym. It's important to be flexible and use your schedule as a guide, not a concrete requirement.

Step 4: Additional Items

When building your calendar, plan for doctor's appointments, car maintenance, your vacation getaway, and other events. Is something coming up that you need to make an alternate plan for? Maybe buying a house or a car will require you to schedule a meeting at the bank during normal bank hours. Maybe your family takes a regular trip to the beach every summer. Make sure not to omit events that only occur periodically. Without looking at the bigger picture, you may forget or have to miss out on important events because you didn't plan far enough in advance.

Step 5: Revise and Repeat

Try out your preliminary schedule for a while. What works well? What doesn't work? One mistake I've made in building calendars and goal lists is being inflexible and not adapting them to how I'm actually spending my time.

You might plan to work out three days a week before heading to your job, only to discover you're not as much of a morning person as you thought. Change your template schedule and work out in the afternoon. There is no right way, and your first attempts may not come up with the best schedule for you.

As a "Type A" pharmacist—the personality type obsessed with achievement, accomplishing tasks quickly, and controlling situations—if I failed to achieve something on my goals list or a preplanned schedule didn't work for me, I'd quickly abandon it altogether rather than make adjustments or change my expectations. Remember that writing something down doesn't bind you. You're giving yourself a starting point from which to base your search for the best schedule.

Box 7-1

Further Reading to Aid Workplace Adjustment

Communication and Work Skills

101 Ways to Improve Your Pharmacy Worklife
(Jacobs MR. Washington, D.C.: American Pharmaceutical Association; 2001.)
This book, by a community pharmacist who has refused to passively accept the status quo during his many years in practice, offers practical tips for reducing stress and improving your professional well-being.

continued on page 102

Box 7-1

continued

Communication Skills for Pharmacists
(Berger BA. 3rd ed. Washington, D.C.: American Pharmacists Association; 2009.)
In this book you'll find practical advice on building relationships with patients and physicians, listening and responding appropriately, effective patient counseling, supportive communication, managing conflict, assertiveness, and more.

Pharmacists Talking with Patients: A Guide to Patient Counseling
(Rantucci MJ. 2nd ed. Philadelphia: Lippincott Williams & Wilkins; 2007.)
Inside this book is an easy-to-understand introduction to patient counseling for pharmacy students and practicing pharmacists. Topics include the therapeutic alliance between health professionals and patients, collaborative working relationships between pharmacists and physicians, and cultural and literacy issues.

Strengths Finder 2.0.
(Rath T. New York: Gallup Press; 2007.)
This is a new and improved version of a book and online assessment tool first released in 2001. You can read the book in one sitting, but it's a great reference for ways to determine your strengths and apply them.

Writing, Speaking, and Communication Skills for Health Professionals
(Barnard S, Hughes KT, St. James D, et al. New Haven, Conn.: Yale University Press; 2001.)
Experts in health care communications provide useful tips for organizing data, writing conference posters and other materials, teaching about science and health care, building a practice, and holding effective meetings. They offer a great overview of the business aspects of health care.

Working with Different Generations

Bridging the Generation Gap: How to Get Radio Babies, Boomers, Gen Xers, and Gen Yers to Work Together and Achieve More
(Gravett L, Throckmorton R. Franklin Lakes, N.J.: Career Press; 2007.)
This engaging book about generational differences in the workplace has an unusual twist. The authors write from two distinct voices, one a Baby Boomer and the other a Generation Xer, in a point-counterpoint style to highlight similarities and differences. It includes hands-on experiences, real-life cases, recommended solutions, and research to help members of any generation better relate to minimize conflict, miscommunication, and wasted energy.

continued on page 103

Box 7-1

continued

Generations at Work: Managing the Clash of Veterans, Boomers, Xers, and Nexters in Your Workplace
(Zemke R, Raines C, Filipczak B. New York: AMACOM; 2000.)
This easy-to-read text is a great introduction to dealing with generational differences in the workplace. Although helpful for anyone, it is particularly geared toward managers or supervisors managing employees of different generations. It includes a chapter about each generation, case studies about generational differences in the workplace, suggested solutions by outside experts, and web resources for further information.

When Generations Collide: Who They Are. Why They Clash. How to Solve the Generational Puzzle at Work
(Lancaster LC, Stillman D. New York: HarperCollins; 2002.)
To help readers improve interactions with coworkers and employees, this book explores how each generation functions in a work environment. It provides tips for managing each generation from recruitment to retention, and guides you in looking for characteristics in future employers that suggest generational differences are celebrated as strengths.

Reducing Error in the Health Care Workplace

Crossing the Quality Chasm: A New Health System for the 21st Century
(Institute of Medicine, Committee on Quality of Health Care in America. Washington, D.C.: National Academies Press; 2001.)
This report describes the gap between care that should be given to patients based on science and research, and the care they actually receive. It recommends sweeping, system-wide changes and also serves to inspire action from pharmacists to improve health care delivery.

Medication Errors
(Cohen M, ed. 2nd ed. Washington, D.C.: American Pharmacists Association; 2007.)
Inside you'll find a detailed description of the causes of medication errors as well as tips for reducing and preventing them. Both new and seasoned pharmacists will find this thorough examination interesting and instructive.

continued on page 104

Box 7-1

continued

Preventing Medication Errors: Quality Chasm Series
(Aspden P, Wolcott J, Bootman JL, et al. Washington, D.C.: National Academies Press; 2007.)
This report examines the incidence and cost of medication errors and recommends action steps for preventing them in the health care workplace. Recognizing potential weaknesses in a system or process helps you see medication errors in a less punitive light, recommend potential solutions, and make useful changes in your work environment.

To Err Is Human: Building a Safer Health System
(Kohn LT, Corrigan JM, Donaldson MS, et al. Washington, D.C.: National Academies Press; 1999.)
Part of a series of publications from the Committee on Quality of Health Care in America, this was one of the first reports to address patient safety and medical errors as systems-based problems. It provides a helpful perspective on the fallibility of health care systems and the inevitability of making mistakes and describes numerous ways to decrease the likelihood of errors.

Holiday Schedules

It may not feel like it sometimes, but most supervisors *want* happy employees, and they do their best to accommodate requests made by their staff. So if you want to take time off for a religious holiday, put in the request as soon as you can. As a manager, I honor as many time-off requests as possible, and I expect my boss to do the same. You may find, if you follow a religious holiday schedule that is less common in your area, that getting time-off approval is relatively easy because you're not competing with everyone else. I can rarely accommodate all the requests I receive for time off at Christmas, so if an employee is able to work on Christmas but needs another day off, it makes approving all the requests easier for me.

Nearly everyone in health care is asked to work a holiday at some point, especially if your area provides direct patient care. It's not fun, but look at it this way—you'd rather be in those shoes than in your patients'. Chances are, when the next holiday rolls around, you'll be at the top of the list for time off. Here are some tips for handling the holidays:

- **Plan Ahead.** So you don't have to miss out on family events, plan holiday gatherings several months in advance and conduct them on a day other than the actual holiday. Think of the holiday as whatever day the family can be together.

— **Invite Loved Ones to Work.** Some health care employers let you invite guests for short visits during holiday shifts.

— **Brace Yourself.** Caring for sick, lonely patients on holidays can be gut-wrenching. Emotions run high during major holidays anyway, but illness and emergencies can be especially tough to cope with. The good thing is, the busier you are, the faster your time on duty passes.

— **Empathize.** Be extra kind to patients rather than taking out your frustration on them. Remember, they don't want to be there either.

— **Enjoy the Perks.** Maybe you get paid more for working on a holiday. Maybe you get a free meal. If your employer doesn't offer these benefits, make the day festive by bringing in homemade dishes to share or organizing a gift exchange.

— **Find a Way to Worship.** It's tough to miss religious ceremonies that can't be replicated before or after the holiday. You can always visit your facility's chapel, meet with a pastoral staff member, or find a quiet spot to pray on your own.

— **Accept Holidays as Part of the Schedule.** If you're lucky, working holidays is an occasional annoyance, but you may have to do it regularly—in which case, just accept it. Attitude is everything. If you can't adjust—or don't find that something else compensates, such as working a great schedule most of the year—it's not the right job for you. As with all things in your workplace environment, handling the situation with professionalism and maturity is the best way to go.

Your First Days on the Job

My top advice, after reading lots of articles and "top 10" lists, is this: exceed expectations. This means dress better than the dress code requires, arrive early, leave late, work hard, and maintain a positive outlook.

Finish Your Homework

You researched your employer during the application and interview stages; now you need to fill in the gaps. Read whatever you can, such as the employee handbook, brochures and marketing materials, the annual report, and internal documents you didn't have access to before you came on board. If someone in your professional network knows an employee at the company, try to meet with the employee before your first day to gain extra insights. You want to understand more completely what the company does and how you fit in.

Dress Professionally

A neat, well-put-together appearance creates a good impression with your new coworkers. Dress a notch above the standard at your workplace. If you look professional, people tend to assume that your work is high quality, too. Planning what you're going to wear each day for the first week of work can make the process less stressful. Start with your most conservative outfits and transition to more casual as appropriate.

Arrive Early, Leave Late

Arriving early and refraining from dashing to the door at the end of the workday conveys the impression that you're enthusiastic and ambitious about your work. Never be late unless there's a real emergency, so people know they can count on you. If you relocated to take this job, plan your route to work as well as some alternates (even if you have a navigation system in your car) to decrease the likelihood that traffic, road construction, or other obstacles will delay you.

Get to Know Your Coworkers

Settling into a new job means becoming part of its social network. You spend more waking hours with coworkers than with most other people, and how they see you can affect both your happiness and your job effectiveness. Don't keep a distance; instead, socialize with your new coworkers over lunch and coffee.

Learn the Culture

Observing and listening are two of the best skills you can use to get a handle on your workplace culture. The information you pick up by paying careful attention can better prepare you for everything from giving a presentation to climbing the career ladder in your organization. Some questions to consider:

- Is your company highly goal-oriented? What about your department or site?
- Are employees expected to develop short-term and long-term goals? What about individual sites or departments?
- How is "success" measured?
- How are requests for time off approved?
- How flexible or laid back is your work environment?
- Who makes the big decisions? What about the small ones?

Meet people in your area and in the departments where you cross paths. Seek out people who have been there a long time and ask for any advice they might be able to offer. Ask lots of questions to understand how things work, including the unwritten rules not covered explicitly in your employer's policies and procedures.

For example, does the first person to arrive for the morning shift always make a fresh pot of coffee? Do people sit in certain places during a particular meeting? How do coworkers typically acknowledge birthdays? Are gifts or cards customary, or are they discouraged? Being aware of the unwritten rules helps you integrate into your work environment more smoothly. That doesn't mean you adopt negative behaviors too—such as showing up 10 minutes late to meetings just because everyone else does.

Ask for Help

You may worry that you'll seem incompetent if you ask for help, but actually, seeking help lets you bond with coworkers and helps you avoid mistakes. You'll learn faster and connect with others better if you reach out when you're unsure about a task or process. But avoid asking the same questions over and over. Take notes to refer to next time.

Take Initiative

The first few weeks on the job, you'll probably be given a lighter workload than your coworkers so you can get up to speed gradually. Let your supervisor know you're ready to add more work as soon as you've mastered what you were originally assigned. The sooner you can handle a full workload, the better the impression you'll make.

Make a Plan

Plot out the things you're expected to learn and some additional goals you set for yourself. Prioritize them to keep you focused on what's most important. Having a plan helps you monitor and achieve your goals during your first few weeks on the job, and also helps you stay motivated. Sharing your plan and your progress with your supervisor will make you seem organized and ambitious.

Communicate with Your Boss

Find out how you and your boss will stay in touch about your priorities and your progress—weekly meetings? Written progress reports? Ask his or her expectations of you and live up to them.

Maintain a Positive Outlook

Optimists usually make better first impressions and are seen more favorably by colleagues and superiors than negative people are. Be friendly and introduce yourself warmly to colleagues you don't know. Smile when you pass coworkers in the hall. Avoid complaining about anything, don't gossip, and refrain from making negative comments about people—especially those you work with.

Working with Others

When I first asked my students what they wanted to know about working with others, they asked how to build successful working relationships with physicians, nurses, technicians, and other pharmacists. I had a hard time developing a distinct set of tips, but then it hit me. The students felt they needed to change their own work habits or do something differently based on the rank, profession, or context of the other person. But you can't make global assumptions about these groups and how they operate.

As a young pharmacist, I quickly learned that not all physicians do things the same way. Some want more information, some less. Some put you on the spot while rounding, others ask your opinion when you're not on the hot seat. Some openly express appreciation for your contributions or see value in multidisciplinary patient care teams. Others don't.

Until now, you probably haven't had to work for extended periods with people who are very different from you. It's human nature to gravitate to people who share our goals, ambitions, outlook on life, interests, and hobbies—and it's easy to do that in school. But in the workplace, you'll be thrown together with people who are less like you and you'll spend *more* time interacting with them. In the long run, it will make you a better communicator, listener, observer, and learner.

Rather than focusing on differences between professional groups, let's look at some other differences in the workplace to help you appreciate and cope with them.

Generational Differences

Four generations fill the workplace right now, and each has a different world view shaped by conditions as they grew up.
- Veterans (or Traditionalists) – Born between 1925 and 1945
- Baby Boomers – Born between 1946 and 1960
- Generation X (or "Xers") – Born between 1961 and 1980
- Generation Y (or "Nexters," "Millennials," "Generation Next") – Born between 1981 and 2000

The unique trends, technological advances, world events, and economic conditions of each generation affect their attitudes, values, and work style. Table 7-1 describes experiences, values, and traits that characterize each generation. Box 7-2 contains tips that may help you communicate with other generations.

Look at the table to see how many characteristics of your generation match your own. Chances are, it's quite a few—yet you are not a carbon copy of everyone else your age. On page 110 are examples of generalizations I came across while research-ing the generations for this book.

Table 7-1

Defining the Generations

	Veterans (Born 1925 to 1945)	Baby Boomers (1946 to 1960)	Generation X or Xers (1961 to 1980)	Millennials or Generation Nexters (1981 to 2000)
Events and Experiences	Great Depression New Deal World War II Korean War	Civil Rights Sexual Revolution Cold War Space travel Assassinations	Challenger Desert Storm Energy Crisis Dot-com Y2K Activism Clinton/Lewinsky	School shootings Oklahoma City Technology Child-focused world
Values and Traits	Hard work Dedication Sacrifice Honor Discipline Conformity	Optimism Team orientation Involvement Personal gratification Personal growth Loyalty Career driven Challenge and choice	Diversity Pragmatism Techno-literacy Fun and informality Self-reliance Fiercely independent Multitask masters Work/life balance	Realism Feel civic duty Confident Achievement oriented Extreme fun Respect for diversity Communal
Work is...	An obligation	An exciting adventure	A difficult challenge A contract	A means to an end Fulfillment
Leadership Style	Directive Command and control	Consensual Collegial	Everyone is the same Challenge others Ask why	Undetermined; more time is needed to know this group's collective leadership style
Interactive Style	Individual	Team player Loves to have meetings	Entrepreneur	Participative
Communications	Formal Memo	In person	Direct Immediate	Email Voice mail
Feedback and Rewards	No news is good news Satisfaction in a job well done	Don't appreciate it Money Title recognition	Sorry to interrupt, but how am I doing? Freedom is the best reward	Whenever I want it, at the push of a button Meaningful work

continued on page 110

Table 7-1

continued

Messages That Motivate	Your experience is respected	You are valued You are needed	Do it your way Forget the rules	You will work with other bright, creative people
Work and Family Life	Ne'er the twain shall meet	No balance Work to live	Balance	Balance

Adapted from:
1. NIH Work/Life Center. What it's like to work with me: generational diversity in office and team environments [videocast]. Available at: http://videocast.nih.gov/Summary.asp?File=12973
2. Hammill G. Mixing and managing four generations of employees. Available at: www.fdu.edu/newspubs/magazine/05ws/generations.htm.

— Veterans tend not to question or challenge authority or the status quo. This may cause confusion and resentment among the GenXers and GenYs who have been taught to speak up.
— GenXers and GenYs may fail to actively listen to Boomers and Veterans, and as a result may miss valuable information and guidance.

There is truth in these generalizations, but they don't represent hard-and-fast characteristics for each person in a generation. People do not always fit into a neat little generationally defined "box," and each of us is so much more than a list of traits we share with others in our age group.

It's helpful to understand generational differences that can lead to problems and misunderstandings. Keep in mind that the goals you and your coworkers are striving to achieve, although by different means, may be very much the same.

Box 7-2

Tips for Communicating with the Generations

Veterans (Traditionalists)
— Tend to be private; don't expect members to share their thoughts immediately.
— Your word is your bond. Focus on words; body language is less important.
— Face-to-face or written communication is preferred.
— Don't waste their time. Value statements should be clear.
— Communicate formally, using titles.
— Schedule a time to connect versus just stopping by.

continued on page 111

Box 7-2

continued

– Appeal to the greater good.
– Appeal to their sense of right and wrong.
– Some members are not comfortable with computer technology, so don't rely on it for communication.

Baby Boomers
– Body language is very important.
– Speak openly and directly and avoid controlling language.
– Respond to questions with thorough answers and expect to be pressed for details.
– Present options to demonstrate flexibility in your thinking.
– Emphasize fairness to all involved.
– Use brainstorming techniques.
– Communicate using face-to-face methods or phone calls.
– Communicate more verbally than electronically.
– When trying to justify a position, refer to the financial bottom line.

Generation X
– Use email as a primary communication tool.
– Keep conversations short and concise.
– Ask them for and provide them with regular feedback.
– Use an informal communication style.
– Stress personal security.
– Stress personal goals.
– Stress the task at hand.
– Prefers to receive advice through someone they consider a mentor.

Generation Y
– Resents being talked down to.
– Prefers email communication.
– Seek their feedback constantly and give them regular feedback and reinforcement.
– Don't take yourself too seriously.
– Communicate using full range of technology, including instant messaging, Internet, DVDs, MP3 players, and texting.
– Focus on outcomes, not protocol.
– Communicate with clear directions.

Adapted from:
1. Stolz J. Communication key to crossing generational gaps. *The Business Ledger.* September 17, 2008. Available at: www.thebusinessledger.com/Home/Archives/CommentaryViewpoints/tabid/86/newsid415/478/Communication-key-to-cross-generational-relationships/Default.aspx
2. Stewart-Gross B. Generational differences – communication guidelines. Ezine Articles. Available at: ezinearticles.com/?Generational-Differences—Communication-Guidelines&id=859386

Personality Differences

In addition to generational differences in the workplace, you'll also encounter differences in personality, communication style, and preferences—characteristics that make us who we are. In a preceptor training class I teach, I encourage new preceptors to take a brief version of the Myers-Briggs Type Indicator (described in Chapter 3, page 23) because we can't fully understand how to interact with others successfully until we know more about ourselves and our preferences.

The MBTI is just one classification system for describing characteristics and strengths. Others include the 16PF (Sixteen Personality Factor Questionnaire), MMPI (Minnesota Multiphasic Personality Inventory), and the DISC (a personality profile assessing dominance, influence, steadiness, and conscientiousness). Taking the MBTI or one of the other assessments helps you understand how you process information and gives you insight into how and why coworkers and supervisors process it differently. Chapter 3 lists further reading on the MBTI and links where you can take an online assessment.

Dealing with Difficult People

It's inevitable that at some point in your career you'll have a colleague, patient, or supervisor whom you find difficult to deal with. If a person rubs you the wrong way there are many things you can try, depending on how troublesome the situation is and how much it interferes with your work. The options described here range from "turning the other cheek" to finding a new job.

- **Forgive.** That's what the Dalai Lama would do. Ask yourself, "What about this situation or person can I seek to understand and forgive?"

- **Wait it out.** An emotionally charged response never gives you the results you want. Take time to cool off.

- **Ask if "being right" matters.** When we bump heads with someone, we may argue out of an impulse to be right and to defend ourselves. Ask yourself if you are being driven by the need to be right—and if so, what you will gain.

- **Don't respond.** Sometimes a person who makes a negative remark or exhibits a difficult attitude is trying to trigger a reaction from you. Don't give them what they want.

- **Stop talking about it**. When a conflict crops up, it's tempting to chew it over with anyone who'll listen. But this approach gives the conflict energy and causes negative feelings to grow deeper. Instead, stop thinking about it and stop telling the story to others.

— **Try on their shoes.** In a conflict, try putting yourself in the other person's position and consider how he or she may see things. Choose to develop compassion.

— **Look for lessons.** What can you take away from the situation to help you grow and become a better person?

— **Become the observer.** Step back and look at the situation with clarity and detachment rather than letting your emotions escalate.

— **Pose two questions.** Ask yourself, "If I don't respond, what's the worst possible result?" And, "If I do respond, what is the worst possible result?" Chances are you'll realize that nothing good will come from reacting.

— **Pour honey.** Try complimenting the other person for something he did well or point out something you learned from him. Be genuine.

— **Express it.** Dump all your negative thoughts onto a piece of scrap paper. Then crumple it into a ball, toss it in the trash—and imagine all your negative energy disappearing with it.

— **Examine yourself.** Are you sure the other person is really the problem? Are you overreacting? Have you had difficulty with the same type of person or actions before? Maybe there's a pattern here and you have hot buttons that are easily pushed—as we all do.

— **Explore the situation with someone you trust.** Brainstorm ways to address the problem and get a trusted advisor's feedback. Be sure not to whine or complain—simply tell your story and examine ways to respond. If you know someone who deals well with your problem person, ask her how she does it to see if adopting her attitude or behavior might work for you.

— **Talk privately with the problem person.** Use "I" messages to focus on the situation rather than accusing the other person (see Box 7-3). Be pleasant and even-handed. The person may not be aware of the impact his words or actions have on you. He may agree to work on the problem—or he may deny it. Try to reach agreement about positive actions going forward.

— **Follow up.** After the initial discussion, assess whether the behavior has improved or gotten worse. Determine whether a follow-up discussion will have any impact and whether you can count on your boss's support if you pursue it.

— **Confront the behavior publicly.** Direct confrontation works well for some people in some situations. Try gentle humor or an exaggerated physical gesture, such as your hand over your heart to suggest you've been wounded.

— **Rally others, carefully.** If other employees have an issue with the difficult person, you can go to your boss as a group to convince him or her that the behavior's impact is significant and is much more than an isolated incident or a personality difference. Be prepared to give specific examples and to state how the behavior prevents you from doing your job. Focus on ways to solve the problem and avoid looking as if you're ganging up on the person.

— **If all else fails, limit access.** Avoid the other person, as long as it doesn't interfere with your work or career. Choose projects and committees he or she is not involved in. In a big company, you might be able to sidestep the person entirely.

— **Worst case: go elsewhere.** If nothing you've tried has worked and your boss is not supportive, leaving your current employment may be the best option. You may think, "But I'm not the employee with the problem. I simply tried to do my job." You're right, but what price are you willing to pay to stay? Unless the good in your situation outweighs the bad, redirect your energy to finding a new position.

Box 7-3

Using "I" Statements

"I" statements are an effective way to express yourself in difficult situations without judging others or putting them on the defensive. The most effective "I" statements focus on feelings rather than thoughts or opinions. Saying "You're mean to say that" is far less productive than "I feel hurt by what you said."

The typical structure of an "I" message is:
— I feel X (say your feeling)
— when you Y (describe the action)
— because Z (say how the action connects to your feeling)

For example, "I feel frustrated when you talk loudly with coworkers while I am trying to counsel a patient, because I can't communicate effectively with the patient and it makes us look unprofessional as a team."

Managing Your Boss

Effective employees take time to understand the needs, perspectives, challenges, and expectations of their boss. They are sensitive to the boss's work style and recognize ways they can build a strong, cooperative relationship. Make sure you know what your boss is trying to accomplish—and if you're not sure, ask. Don't make assumptions.

"Managing the boss" doesn't mean manipulating him or her—it's simply shaping the relationship in a way that benefits both of you. Here's a list of key pointers for effectively working with your boss.

Control Collaborative Decision-Making

Your boss has many projects and responsibilities to keep tabs on besides yours. Make it easy for him or her when you are discussing status and seeking input on a decision.

- To start, test the waters with your boss to understand the types of decisions you should make on your own and which ones should be made jointly.
- Remind your boss where you left off last time you met and recap the objectives before rushing to the "why" and "how."
- Quickly summarize the options considered and your criteria for selecting the one you are presenting. Focus on points where you need your boss's help. Use graphics and visuals when possible to aid discussion.
- Be prepared with facts and data for your position as well as alternative options. Mention potential outcomes and how you will manage results that are suboptimal.
- After a meeting, summarize the discussion and action items briefly in writing to ensure mutual understanding.
- Do not say critical things to others about decisions you and your boss have made. If you want other opinions, don't go over your boss's head; instead, ask if you can seek input from other administrators and explain the benefit of doing so.

Manage Your Boss's Time

There's only a finite amount of time in a day and everyone seems to have too much to do, including your boss. Anything you can do to add efficiency will be a plus.

- Prepare for meetings in advance and know what you want to accomplish during your time with your boss. Focus on the central issue; spend less time on simpler problems.
- Summarize and synthesize information and options for your boss.
- For large projects, book a series of meetings in advance for different phases, such as talking about research sources, presenting a draft and getting comments, going over a revision, and so on. This way you carve out time you need before your boss's calendar is full.
- Remember, the problems you bring to your boss may represent only 1% of what he or she has to deal with, so don't act as if it's 100%.

Provide Information Effectively

Keeping your boss informed is critical, particularly regarding issues within your areas of responsibility. Managers need to know the status of key efforts and should never be blindsided when it comes to problems or setbacks.

- Avoid information overload. Be selective and distill ideas and problems down to key elements.
- When presenting information that you feel strongly about, especially ideas that may not be well received, omit your emotions and personal feelings and present only facts, data, and information.
- Use your boss's language and look for a spin that aligns your goals with those of your boss without misrepresenting facts or information.
- Share successes—give your boss good news in addition to bad news.
- As much as you can, participate in your boss's information network by interacting with the same people and attending some of the same meetings and presentations. Seek opportunities for two-way communication with your boss in group settings.

Handle Problems Professionally

The emotional dynamics in the workplace can be a lot like those of a family. Be aware of your behavior patterns to avoid lapsing into unproductive ways. Don't let subconscious emotions from past experiences influence your interactions with your supervisor.

- Focus on solutions, not problems. If you need your boss's help with a problem, be prepared to suggest ways of solving it.
- Let your boss know which parts of the problem-solving process you specifically need assistance with.
- Include your manager's goals when presenting problems, ideas, and potential solutions. Attaching a sense of value or priority to the item helps him or her see that resolving it is critical and gets it on the boss's agenda.
- Center the discussion on the organization and its goals rather than on you and your issues.

Promises, Timelines, and Responsibilities

It's natural that you want to please your boss. Sometimes that desire can backfire if you're not realistic about workload and deadlines or if you do not openly communicate with your boss about progress, issues, and obstacles.

- Do not promise what you can't deliver.
- If you cannot meet a timeline, alert your boss ahead of time to prevent bad surprises.
- Check and finalize facts, documentation, memos, and spelling to avoid time spent correcting mistakes and revising information when meeting with your boss.
- Don't shirk responsibility—but at the same time, don't take on something you know nothing about simply to gain your boss's admiration or approval.

- Clarify your boss's expectations of you repeatedly.
- Don't back your boss into a corner; avoid putting him or her in a situation that is embarrassing or difficult to get out of.

Manage Your Differences

Study your boss's style, temperament, and preferences so you know the best way to present information, get approval, and resolve conflicts. Take personal responsibility for making your relationship work—be proactive rather than leaving it up to your boss.

- Observe interactions between your boss and someone with whom your boss interacts well to develop skills in dealing with him or her.
- Clarify your boss's goals and objectives, and understand his or her problems and concerns.
- Understand your mutual need: you need your boss for making connections with the rest of the organization, setting priorities, and obtaining clinical resources, and your boss needs cooperation, reliability, and honesty from you.
- Consider it part of your responsibility to make your boss look good and be successful.
- Appreciate and praise your boss appropriately, but in moderation, to avoid "kissing up."
- Speak your boss's language to get your points across; don't expect him or her to learn yours.
- Gather information from sources your boss uses and trusts: literature, media, and organizational experts.
- Solicit feedback often to avoid being caught off guard by differences in your impression and your boss's impression of your performance.
- Don't expect your boss to change. Work on understanding your own behavior to have a better relationship. If you want your boss to use a specific positive behavior, such as active listening, model that behavior in your interactions.
- Don't talk poorly about your boss in front of others.

Communicate

To work effectively with your boss, you need to understand how he or she likes to receive information. Some managers are more visual, some more interactive. Some like written reports and others prefer quick verbal updates. Does your boss like email, phone, or face-to-face? Graphics? Bullet points? Can you use instant messaging and texting in certain situations?

- Rather than presenting ideas as you would like them presented to you, present them in the way that meets your supervisor's needs.
- Don't assume your boss won't appreciate your taking the initiative to educate him or her; no one can stay on top of all news and developments.
- Help your boss gain buy-in and support for his or her endeavors with your colleagues and direct reports.

- Be respectful of your boss, but not scared. Maintain rapport and treat your boss as a friend in social and organizational gatherings.
- Use "default communication" when appropriate to move a project forward (such as "I will submit this article for publication unless I hear from you otherwise"). This method prevents you from waiting for permission when something is time-sensitive and you know your boss may be bogged down.
- Constantly consider word choice in interactions with and in front of your boss, and maintain a positive tone.

Tips for Developing Self-Confidence

Students whom I precept often ask me about self-confidence. They wonder, "How can I be confident without the safety nets I had as a student?" Or "How can I trust myself now that I am the one making final decisions?" They worry about how to assert themselves as knowledgeable professionals—what if people see them as young or incompetent? And how can they maintain a professional image when they are still seeking help and answers themselves? These basic tips will help you work on building your confidence.

Start by being grateful for what you have, rather than focusing on the chase for new things you think will make you happy. Learn who you are, recognize your values, understand what you want your life to be like in the future, and be true to yourself.

Spend Time with Confident People

Surround yourself with positive people and seek the company of those who exhibit confidence. Their energy and inner strength will inspire you. You can model your behavior after theirs. You will feel more empowered just by listening to them talk. And you can ask them for tips to take your confidence to the next level. Surely all pharmacists have felt doubts or trepidation at times—how did they cope and get past it?

Find Mentors

Nearly all successful people have a mentor—someone who has already done what you are working toward and who is willing to offer advice and coaching. Having a good mentor—or several—is one of the best ways to grow and succeed quickly. Not only do you get great tips, but having an accomplished professional believe in you is a real confidence booster.

I began selecting mentors early in my career, looking for people whose practices or communication styles I admired, as well as those demonstrating devotion to health care or pharmacy. These mentors—excellent leaders, clinicians, and teachers—have been influential in making me the professional I am today.

What I failed at was selecting an arsenal of mentors who are experts in several different areas, such as work/life balance, financial planning, and so on. Chapter 10 covers more about choosing mentors, and being one.

Understand It's Only a Feeling

A good way to become confident is to act as if you are confident. Over time it becomes a habit. Smile and stand up straight. Work on your relaxation skills, too. Think of a situation where you felt confident. Relive it in your head, imagining all the details, including the tingling in your muscles, the steady beat of your heart.

Think of how someone you admire exhibits confidence. What does she say? How does she hold herself? How does she treat people? Incorporate these traits into your own behavior and tap into that confident feeling you have known before.

Remember, however, that confidence without competence is a dangerous combination. In that case, it becomes arrogance—which is something to avoid. Review Table 7-2, The Learning Matrix, to recognize levels of competence in skills. It is normal for your confidence to grow as your competence increases. Only at level 1—where you don't know that you don't know—is your confidence most likely to be out of sync with your competence.

List Reasons to Be Confident

Write down all your successes, skills, qualities, and goals. List 50 reasons why you can be confident today, and include everything that pops into your mind. This list reinforces the concept that you are confident and helps you see yourself that way more consistently.

Focus on Achievements and Strengths

Did you ever see Stuart Smalley, the fictional character performed by Al Franken on *Saturday Night Live*, reminding himself, "I'm good enough, I'm smart enough, and doggone it, people like me"? It's a humorous take on a real truth—focusing on your strengths rather than your shortcomings builds confidence. Keep the items on your list (above) in the forefront of your mind. If you find yourself thinking about how you failed, also look at what you managed to do right and how you could do better next time.

Make a Declaration

Tell someone whose opinion you value that you will be confident at a particular event. Your desire to impress this person will help you be at your very best. And when you demand more of yourself you'll be amazed at what you can do.

Prepare and Practice

Have you watched an athlete or performer in action and noticed how easy he or she makes it look? It's because they practice endlessly and they build their confidence every day. When you invest time to hone your skills, you recognize that you'll perform when the curtain goes up. You can never be over-trained or over-skilled for any challenge in life.

Table 7-2

The Learning Matrix

Level 1 Unconscious Incompetence	You Don't Know That You Don't Know	At this level you are blissfully ignorant: you have a complete lack of knowledge and skills in the subject in question. On top of this, you are unaware of this lack of skill, and your confidence may therefore far exceed your abilities.
Level 2 Conscious Incompetence	You Know That You Don't Know	At this level you find there are skills you need to learn, and you may be shocked to discover that others are much more competent than you. As you realize that your ability is limited, your confidence drops. You go through an uncomfortable period as you learn these new skills when others are much more competent and successful than you are.
Level 3 Conscious Competence	You Know That You Know	At this level you acquire the new skills and knowledge. You put your learning into practice and you gain confidence in carrying out the tasks or jobs involved. You are aware of your new skills and work on refining them. You are still concentrating on the performance of these activities, but as you get more practice and experience, these become increasingly automatic.
Level 4 Unconscious Competence	You Don't Know That You Know. It Just Seems Easy!	At this level your new skills become habits, and you perform the task without conscious effort and with automatic ease. This is the peak of your confidence and ability.
Adapted from: www.mindtools.com/pages/article/newISS_96.htm		

Set Goals and Reward Yourself

Learn to set reachable goals for yourself and break difficult tasks into smaller steps. When you achieve goals, reward yourself! The reward doesn't have to be big, costly, or time-consuming, but it's important to acknowledge your achievements, even to yourself, as you climb the ladder to well-developed confidence.

Making Mistakes

Everyone makes mistakes. It's a common saying—and it's true, we all do. Usually we can correct our errors or just forget about them and move on. But making a mistake in health care can be serious, especially if it affects a patient.

Luckily, many of us work in environments where errors are described as failures of the system, rather than failures of the individual. If the correct checks and balances are in place, it takes multiple errors by multiple health care professionals for a mistake to reach, much less harm, a patient. Here are some tips to help you avoid and deal with mistakes.

Plan for Prevention

Wherever you work, make sure that the appropriate systems, processes, checks, and balances are in place to prevent errors from occurring. If you are unclear about a process, unsure about a dosage, unfamiliar with a medication, or otherwise concerned with a situation, ask a colleague for a second opinion or look up additional information. In fact, I recommend asking a colleague *and* looking it up.

Don't Assume It'll Never Happen to You

A supervisor once told me he had never made a mistake. It's easier for me to believe he'd won the lottery. I think what he meant was he wasn't *aware* of making any mistakes. The real problem is whether, when all is said and done, an error actually occurs. I guarantee you that I've pulled the wrong drug off the shelf while dispensing—even in the last month. Does that make me a bad pharmacist? No. Does it mean I'm incompetent? No.

If the system is working properly, with its associated checks and balances, the technician who counts the tablets will alert me to the situation. If the technician misses it, the other pharmacist on duty will discover the problem once the prescription reaches the check-off station. When the issue *is* brought to my attention, I don't brush it off. *Phew! Crisis averted.* I remind myself that situations like this are the reason for the checks and balances. It can and will happen to you.

Take Responsibility

If an error does occur, take responsibility. Inform the patient, caregiver, health care provider, or other necessary individuals. Assess the risk of harm or the potential untoward effects. Notify the appropriate personnel, including your supervisor and others within your organization who need to be aware of the error. Your organization may have a policy or procedure for error reporting you can refer to.

Just because you take responsibility for an error doesn't mean you're admitting guilt or otherwise indemnifying yourself. In fact, the error may have occurred when you weren't on the clock. It doesn't excuse you from having to deal with the situation. The system failed and you are the one who must repair things as best as you can. Be professional and mature, and employ communication skills discussed earlier in this chapter.

Don't Beat Yourself Up

Apology is necessary; blame and guilt are not. You did not personally cause this error all on your own. In fact, if you are the sole cause of this incident, I'd argue there's something wrong with the system in which you are working and it needs to be fixed—fast! Don't believe me? Read some of the recommended texts in Box 7-1 to learn more.

Document

Chances are your institution has a system in place for documenting errors. If not, be sure to document, using the Food and Drug Administration's MedWatch Reporting Form. (You can download the form at www.fda.gov.)

And be sure the error is followed up and investigated properly. An action plan should be developed to identify processes or procedures that need to be modified to prevent this situation from occurring again.

Learn from the Error

Even if you are not the one responsible for the action plan or investigation, consciously look for things you can do to prevent an error like this one from recurring. And whenever you have a *"Phew! Crisis averted"* moment, ask yourself: Was I going too fast? Not paying attention? Do I need to refocus or do things a different way? Even if the error had no consequences, it's still important to reflect on what you might have done differently. And then move on. No wallowing in guilt, losing sleep, or otherwise punishing yourself.

Taking Charge of Your Career and Honing Your Skills

"Pharmacy needs many different kinds of leaders to complete the transition to a patient-focused profession. We critically need leadership in practice innovation. The most effective leaders know their strengths and follow their passion."

—Lucinda L. Maine, executive vice president and CEO, American Association of Colleges of Pharmacy

It takes months, years, even a lifetime to master the skills covered in this chapter. You can't get started too soon. Being a professional means constantly learning and growing. Everyone always has room for improvement! The advice, tips, and resources that follow should help you take charge of your career and develop skills you need along the way.

Leadership

Pharmacists need to build leadership skills, even if they're not planning to pursue careers in management or administration, because such skills are part of being an effective health care professional. What's the difference between "leadership skills" and "management skills"? Here's a clue from *Leadership as a Professional Obligation: Report from the Student New Practitioner Leadership Task Force*, published in July 2009:

"A 'management' course in pharmacy school curricula may prepare students to assemble a basic budget but might leave out lessons on the communication and consensus-building skills needed to ensure that the budget is adopted."

Because most schools of pharmacy don't incorporate much leadership training into the Doctor of Pharmacy degree curriculum, I've provided these suggestions.

Understand the Problem

If you refer to the Learning Matrix in Chapter 7 (see page 120), right now you're probably at Level 1 when it comes to leadership skills—and it's time to move to Level 2. Start by reading the *Leadership as a Professional Obligation* report mentioned above, which talks about a "pharmacy leadership crisis" and the difficulties in filling pharmacy director positions today.

You can find the report on the website of the American Society of Health-System Pharmacists (ASHP) Foundation at www.ashpfoundation.org. It was developed by the Student New Practitioner Leadership Task Force, which was established in 2007 to address:

— The level of students' and new practitioners' exposure to leadership concepts in their studies or practice settings.
— Specific gaps in leadership education and training and innovative ways to address these gaps.
— Opportunities to incorporate leadership education into pharmacists' training.
— Values, issues, and challenges that influence new practitioners' desire or ability to assume leadership roles.

Pharmacists must have leadership skills to motivate patients to stick with their medication regimens, to educate nurses about proper administration, and to guide physicians on appropriate prescribing. The report gives specific recommendations, such as urging employers to establish programs for developing leadership skills and to require mandatory competency assessments on leadership.

Another good source for understanding leadership issues is *A Force for Change: How Leadership Differs from Management* by John P. Kotter, one of the great leadership gurus of our day. He discusses why leadership is rarely associated with larger-than-life charisma, how leadership is different from management, and why both are essential for business success. He notes that:

— Thousands of companies are over managed and under led.
— Leadership is a process that creates change.
— Many executives lack an understanding of what leadership is.
— It can take many leaders and managers working together to launch common-sense ideas and procedures for top results.

See Box 8-1 for other recommended readings on leadership.

Learn from Those Who Came Before You

To get inspired, look for examples of leaders in your everyday life—not just in your profession or studies but in other fields and locations—and read about leaders whose paths you might never cross. During my residency, I mentioned to my residency director that I had a desire to learn more about leadership. He told me to read one Harvey A. K. Whitney Award Lecture each week and come prepared to discuss what I'd learned. This award, established in 1950, recognizes outstanding contributors to hospital pharmacy, and each winner gives a lecture. (You can find the lectures at www.harveywhitney.org/lectures.)

Box 8-1

Selected Reading on Leadership

General

The 8th Habit: From Effectiveness to Greatness
(Covey SR. New York: Free Press; 2004.)
To thrive, innovate, excel, and lead in what Covey calls the "New Knowledge Worker Age," you must find your voice and inspire others to find theirs. The 8th habit involves finding a new mind set, a new skill set, and a new tool set to achieve personal and organizational excellence.

The 12 Elements of Great Managing
(Wagner R, Harter JK. New York: Gallup Press; 2006.)
How do great managers inspire top performance, generate enthusiasm, unite disparate personalities, and drive teams to achieve higher goals? This book follows great managers and their teams in efforts to turn around a failing call center, save a struggling hotel, improve patient care in a hospital, and deal with other challenges. The book draws on interviews with 10 million employees and managers in 114 countries as well as recent discoveries in neuroscience, game theory, psychology, sociology, and economics.

The Five Dysfunctions of a Team
(Lencioni P. San Francisco: Jossey-Bass; 2002.)
This instructive leadership fable looks at the complex world of teams, reminding us that leadership requires as much courage as it does insight. The author explores five dysfunctions at the heart of why teams, even the best ones, often struggle, and outlines steps to overcome these problems.

Good to Great: Why Some Companies Make the Leap...And Others Don't
(Collins JC. New York: HarperBusiness; 2001.)
Based on the results of a five-year study, *Good to Great* examines universal characteristics that take a company from good to great. The research team used tough benchmarks to identify 28 companies that leapt to great results and sustained those results for at least 15 years. Determinants of greatness that the book discusses include type of leadership, a culture that combines discipline with entrepreneurship, making the most of what the company does well, and avoiding pitfalls of radical-change programs and restructurings.

continued on page 126

Box 8-1

continued

Leadership and Self-Deception: Getting Out of the Box
(The Arbinger Institute. San Francisco: Berrett-Koehler; 2000.)
The authors use a compelling story to examine the premise that leaders can overcome self-deception to become a consistent catalyst of success. The key to leadership lies deeper than any technique, behavior, or skill—it has to do with being honest, straightforward, and genuine.

The Leadership Challenge
(Kouzes JM, Posner BZ. 4th ed. San Francisco: Jossey-Bass; 2007.)
After 20 years in print and three editions, this text continues to be a premier resource on becoming a leader. It includes the latest research and case studies and new stories of real people achieving extraordinary results. The authors talk about "five practices" and "10 commitments" that have been proven by many dedicated, successful leaders.

Leadership from the Inside Out: Becoming a Leader for Life
(Cashman K. 2nd ed. San Francisco: Berrett-Koehler Publishers; 2008.)
This book's core premise is that developing as a whole leader requires developing as a whole person. "We lead by virtue of who we are," the book notes, exploring the areas you must master to influence others and create enduring value. Through illustrative stories and tools, the book emphasizes building awareness, commitment, and practice.

On Becoming a Leader
(Bennis W. 4th ed. New York: Basic Books; 2009.)
Leaders are not born—they are made, according to Bennis, who delves into qualities that define leadership, people who exemplify it, and strategies anyone can apply to achieve it. This classic work has provided insights to countless readers.

On Leadership
(Gardner J. New York: Free Press; 1993.)
In this brilliant examination of how leadership is practiced in America today, Gardner insists that most skills for being an effective leader can be learned. Drawing from his vast experience in government, corporate, and nonprofit sectors, he notes that leaders must be committed to lifelong personal growth, renewing values and institutions, building community, and releasing human potential.

continued on page 127

Box 8-1

continued

Synchronicity: The Inner Path of Leadership

(Jaworski J. San Francisco: Berrett-Koehler Publishers; 1996.)
Leadership is not about positional power or accomplishments, the author argues, but is about creating a domain in which people continually learn and become more capable of participating in their unfolding future. Shaping this future calls for three basic shifts of mind—in how you see the world, understand relationships, and make commitments.

Your Leadership Legacy

(Galford RM, Maruca RF. Boston: Harvard Business School; 2006.)
Based on stories of top leaders who have shaped successful careers, the book explores the art of "legacy thinking," helping you to formulate a legacy that will exert a positive effect on your work immediately. Your legacy is defined by how others approach work and life as a result of having worked with you, including time management, project management, and people management.

Specific to Pharmacy

The Conscience of a Pharmacist: Essays on Vision and Leadership for the Profession

(Zellmer WA. Bethesda, Md.: American Society of Health-System Pharmacists; 2002.)
The essays in this book, first published as editorials in the *American Journal of Health-System Pharmacy,* offer historical perspective and insights into how pharmacists have worked to make pharmacy a better profession.

Harvey A. K. Whitney Award Lectures

(The ASHP Research and Education Foundation. Available at: www.harveywhitney.org)
The Harvey A. K. Whitney Lecture Award is given annually to someone who has made significant contributions to health-system pharmacy. Each recipient gives a lecture containing leadership insights and advice.

Heroes of Pharmacy: Professional Leadership in Times of Change

(Worthen DB. Washington, D.C.: American Pharmacists Association; 2007.)
Examine key issues by reading about the lives and careers of those who dealt with these issues. The book includes essays on the professional lives of 28 pharmacy statesmen, reformers, activists, educators, ethicists, editors, and pioneers and provides insights into two centuries of professional progress in education, community and institutional practice, manufacturing, government, publishing, association leadership, and military service.

continued on page 128

Box 8-1

continued

Leadership and Advocacy for Pharmacy
(Boyle CJ, Beardsley RS, Holdford DA, eds. Washington, D.C.: American Pharmacists Association; 2007.)
This book discusses the elements of effective leadership by covering relevant theories and their application to real experiences, including effective techniques, mistakes made, and integrating leadership into everyday life. Each chapter focuses on a specific aspect of leadership or advocacy in pharmacy.

I learned so much from this simple exercise of "read and reflect" that I suggest you develop a similar plan for yourself, whether a mentor is willing to discuss the lectures with you or not. For example, some points that stood out for me:
– Each of us is individually responsible for our own pharmacy legacy, as James C. McAllister III noted in 2003. He described the principles of legacy in detail: caring, honesty and integrity, attitude, commitment, leadership, and stewardship.
– In his 1985 lecture, Fred M. Eckel said that "rather than concerning ourselves with the whole problem, we need to focus on the part we can control" when we get discouraged by looking at what needs to be done in the profession of pharmacy.
– Marianne F. Ivey focused on the importance of being able to change, grow, and adapt to our success as pharmacists in her 1993 lecture.

Seek Additional Education

Following this step was one of the best decisions I made when developing my leadership skills. I had already completed school and residency training and was beginning my pharmacy career when I found out about a distance-learning program at the Ohio State University School of Pharmacy called the Latiolais Leadership Program. I decided to enroll, and I received tuition assistance from both my state pharmacy association and my employer. This is one option for you, among others.

If you're still in school, your program may offer leadership skills training or certificate programs. If you're past that point, your employer may even provide some training opportunities. For example, the institution where I work, New Hanover Regional Medical Center, has the Leadership Development Institute designed by the Studer Group. Below is a listing of leadership programs that may be appropriate for you.

The Ohio State University Latiolais Leadership Program
This program offers the online Essence of Leadership Course, which combines self-assessment, assigned self-study, interactive discussion questions, assignments,

projects, and a final examination. It consists of six classes, each of which is to be completed during one month. The classes cover:
- Becoming a leader, including individual leadership styles
- Communication and personal skills
- Leading and managing change
- Using networks, influence, and negotiation
- Building teams and relationships, mentoring, and succession planning
- Pharmaceutical leadership

This program is open to anyone interested, but was specifically designed for aspiring pharmacy leaders seeking to improve their leadership competencies. More information can be obtained at http://pharmacy.osu.edu/latiolais/index.cfm.

ASHP Foundation Pharmacy Leadership Academy

Designed as a comprehensive curriculum to enhance the leadership and management skills of new and aspiring pharmacy leaders, the Academy's program runs its academic year from January through November. Sponsored by the American Society of Health-System Pharmacists Foundation, the Academy offers nine modules, each to be completed in one month, led by content experts who serve as the Academy faculty members in a distance-learning format. The modules are:
- Leading the Pharmacy Enterprise
- Providing Leadership in Safety and Quality
- Understanding Information Technology and Systems
- Leading People
- Leadership for Effective Financial Management
- Leading Change and Innovation
- Leading for Results
- Gaining Leadership Skills through Self-Development
- Building Presence with Executive Leadership

This program is open to anyone interested, but was specifically designed to enhance the leadership and management skills of new and aspiring pharmacy leaders. More information, including a downloadable application, can be obtained at www.ashpfoundation.org.

Annual ASHP Conference for Leaders in Health-System Pharmacy

A two-day meeting for all levels of managers, seasoned practitioners, new supervisors, and pharmacy residents, this program includes interactive workshops, how-to discussions, and intensive sessions that look in depth at a particular topic. An application is not required; simply sign up and pay a registration fee, much like other meetings held by national pharmacy associations. Find more information at www.ashpadvantage.com/leaders.

ACCP Leadership and Management Certificate Program

This educational program from the American College of Clinical Pharmacy is designed for those currently in or aspiring to leadership or management positions. It involves 28 contact hours of live, in-class experience obtained in conjunction with ACCP's spring and annual meetings, as well as outside readings and online portfolio-based assignments. After you finish the requirements, ACCP provides an official certificate of completion. Find more information at www.accp.com.

Self-Directed Learning

Develop a simple plan for self-directed learning and take advantage of the many excellent leadership texts available, both general and pharmacy-specific (see Box 8-1 for suggestions). To create a list of topics to learn about, look at those listed above under "Seek Additional Education." In general, key topics to explore as you build leadership skills include communication, conflict resolution, decision making, consensus building, vision and focus, promoting teamwork, and motivating others.

Management Skills

Although good managers often exercise good leadership skills and good leaders often demonstrate good management skills, the two are not the same. In this section we'll talk about management in terms of "what is being managed." You draw on different skills—with some overlap—for managing time, projects, and people.

Time Management

If you don't use your time wisely, you can never get it back. How often do you feel as if there's too much to do and not enough time? Good time management is essential for career success, allowing you to be productive, deliver what you promise, accomplish more with less effort, and keep stress under control.

Use Time Management Tools

In the article "Time Management Tips" in the September 1997 issue of *The Consultant Pharmacist,* author Jeannette Wick suggests using planning grids, "one of the best tools for organizing your workload and making sure routine tasks are performed, and performed on time," she says. She uses a 12-month planning grid to monitor completion of responsibilities on her facility's pharmacy and therapeutics committee—however, there are many different types of planning grids. Figure 8-1, for example, shows a grid for breaking a larger project into weekly and daily increments. The grid in Figure 8-2 is organized by topic, with tasks assigned to specific people and due dates clearly spelled out.

Other helpful tools include:
- Prioritized to-do lists, on which you cross off items as they're completed.
- Preformatted data entry forms for collecting and analyzing data—particularly helpful for tasks such as drug utilization reviews.
- Spreadsheet software such as Microsoft Excel, which can be used to organize, sort, and analyze information.
- Self-addressed email messages reminding yourself to complete certain tasks.
- An alarm clock or watch to remind yourself of appointment times, meetings, and deadlines.
- A personal digital assistant (PDA) device, such as a pocket PC or other electronic organizer with or without alarm features.

Build In Relaxation
Schedule breaks at regular times so you get a chance to clear your mind and move around. When you have breaks scheduled, you're more likely to really apply yourself the rest of the time. And take breaks when you need them to avoid the buildup of stress. Go for a short walk or do quick stretches.

Figure 8-1

Planning Grid Organized by Weeks and Days

Week	Dates	Monday	Tuesday	Wednesday	Thursday	Friday	Saturday	Sunday
Week 1								
Week 2								
Week 3								
Week 4								
Week 5								
Week 6								

Figure 8-2

Planning Grid Organized by Projects

Topic	Discussion	Action	Person Responsible	Due Date
Topic/Project 1				
Topic/Project 2				
Topic/Project 3				
Topic/Project 4				
Topic/Project 5				
Topic/Project 6				

Get plenty of exercise and sleep so you come to work refreshed and function efficiently. When your body and mind are rested, you can complete tasks in less time.

Concentrate

Keep away distractions that drain your productivity. If you're spending too much time on the phone, keep an egg timer at your desk and hold calls to a reasonable limit. If you have an office, close your door when you need to focus.

Schedule your toughest work for the time of day when you tend to be sharpest and most productive. Work methodically and avoid rushing, which boosts the chance of errors. Doing it right the first time is quicker than having to go back and correct something.

Organize

It's easier to get tasks done if your work area is organized. Set aside 10 to 15 minutes each week to clear out junk mail, old papers, and other clutter. Change habits that lead to messes. Keep cleaning supplies handy so you can tidy your workplace while you're on the phone or when a few free seconds crop up. If you have a bit more time, clean out a drawer or part of a filing cabinet. Group certain kinds of tasks, such as ordering or filing, rather than switching back and forth.

For a large task with many facets, break it into pieces so it's not overwhelming. You could sort a stack of papers one day and process a portion each day after that until the task is done. Look at how you accomplish tasks to see if any steps can be eliminated from a process. Maybe you don't need to keep multiple copies or enter data more than once.

Don't Procrastinate

Identify tasks you put off and ask yourself why. Some people avoid tasks they don't feel they do well, so ask for help if you're not sure how to do something. Stop avoiding minor, less important tasks and instead knock off a few while you're on hold or listening to a conference call. Set aside a few minutes each morning for chores like reviewing and deleting email or putting papers in folders. Don't put off dealing with problems of employees and colleagues that end up on your plate—the more time passes, the larger they seem.

Delegate

Don't try to do everything yourself. If someone else is willing to take over a task, let them—even if they're likely to do it differently than you would. For large, tedious tasks, recruit others to help—like emptying a wall of file cabinets or doing an inventory. With frequent breaks, snacks, and conversation, everyone will have fun.

Say No

Use your time and talents wisely and avoid spreading yourself too thin. Stick to accomplishing tasks that are most important to you, your boss, and your organization. When you're asked to do things that do not fit those goals, say no politely. If you'd really like to do what's being asked but don't have time, say, "I can't do this, but I *can*..." and mention a lesser commitment you can make.

Ask the Experts

If someone always seems to be ahead of the game or has a faster way of getting something done, watch, learn, and copy what they do. Ask others how they organize and execute tasks that take you a long time; maybe you've overlooked shortcuts. You can also take a time management course at a local community college or through a seminar group to get tried-and-true tips. Box 8-2 contains a list of recommended reading on time management.

Box 8-2

Recommended Reading on Time Management

- **The 7 Habits of Highly Effective People.** Covey SR. Rev. ed. New York: FreePress/ Simon & Schuster; 2004.
- **The 12 Elements of Great Managing.** Wagner R, Harter JK. New York: Gallup Press; 2006.
- **Achieving Objectives Made Easy! Practical Goal Setting Tools & Proven Time Management Techniques.** Le Blanc R. Maarheeze, The Netherlands: Cranendonck Coaching; 2008.
- **First Things First.** Covey SR, Merrill AR, Merrill RR. London: Simon & Schuster UK Ltd; 1999.
- **Getting Things Done: The Art of Stress-Free Productivity.** Allen D. New York: Viking; 2001.
- **How to Get Control of Your Time and Your Life.** Lakein A. New York: David McKay Co; 1973.
- **Make Every Minute Count: More Than 700 Tips and Strategies That Will Revolutionize How You Manage Your Time.** Lane H, Wayser C. New York: Marlowe & Co; 2000.
- **Management Time: Who's Got the Monkey?** Oncken W, Wass DL. *Harvard Business Review.* November/December 1974;75-80.
- **The Now Habit: A Strategic Program for Overcoming Procrastination and Enjoying Guilt-Free Play.** Fiore NA. Redesigned ed. New York: Tarcher/Penguin Group; 2007.
- **Time Management.** Fleming I. 5th ed. Alresford, England: Management Pocketbooks Ltd; 2003.
- **Time Management from the Inside Out: The Foolproof System for Taking Control of Your Schedule—and Your Life.** Morgenstern J. 2nd ed. New York: Henry Holt; 2004.
- **Working Efficiently.** White SJ. *Am J Health Syst Pharm.* Aug 2007; 64:1587-91.

Project Management

A common saying, "Plan the work and work the plan," gets to the heart of good project management: careful planning. And central to good planning is setting effective short-term goals to help you monitor and control the plan's execution.

A useful approach for setting project management goals is conveyed by the acronym "SMART."

S – Specific
M – Measurable
A – Attainable
R – Relevant
T – Timely

Writing goals that include SMART criteria increases the likelihood that you'll achieve the goals and that you'll be able to demonstrate your success in a concrete and specific way. Some employers' performance evaluation programs require SMART goals because it's simple to assess whether they've been attained. Table 8-1 defines the qualities of SMART goals.

Table 8-1

The Qualities of SMART Goals

S	Specific Goals are:	Described using action verbs Concrete
M	Measurable Goals are:	Descriptive Numeric Quantity/quality
A	Attainable Goals are:	Feasible Appropriately limited in scope Within your control and influence
R	Relevant Goals are:	Important to you, your boss, your employer, your organization, and/or your institution
T	Timely Goals include:	A target date or timeframe Interim steps A plan to monitor progress

The goal "become a licensed pharmacist" is a SMART goal only when you expand it like this: "Become a licensed, practicing pharmacist in the state of North Carolina by passing all exams required by the North Carolina Board of Pharmacy by July 1 of this year."

Another example is "Help my patients with diabetes better manage their disease." When you incorporate SMART criteria, the goal reads: "By October 2010, begin a pharmacist-run diabetes management service at my community pharmacy focused on improving patients' A1c levels and their therapies' compliance with American Diabetes Association criteria over baseline."

Of course, both examples could be broken down further into more specific goals. You can even establish a schedule to ensure that the smaller components of a larger goal (like starting a pharmacist-run diabetes management service) are accomplished in a timely fashion.

If you break down larger project goals, you can apply the SMART goal approach to the subgoals. The key is to write goals that are important and achievable, and that you can accomplish in a specific, predefined time period. And when you meet your goals, you have clear-cut results to demonstrate your success.

People Management

At some point, whether you plan to be a manager or not, you'll find yourself overseeing the work of others—such as technicians, students, colleagues, or employees. You may be a team leader on a project or coordinator of an event that other people are contributing to. You'll need to lead, motivate, and encourage them. And if you teach or precept, you'll need to manage and promote students' learning.

Supervision

Supervision can be tough, even for seasoned pharmacists. An excellent resource is *Supervision: A Pharmacy Perspective* by Jeannette Y. Wick (listed in Box 8-3), which covers many topics helpful to new supervisors such as supervising former peers, mistakes supervisors make, lessons for new supervisors, expectations, how to hire, performance evaluations, and learning to motivate others. Four key functions of supervisors are defined below.

- **Planning** is the process of setting goals, developing strategies, and outlining tasks and schedules to accomplish those goals.
- **Controlling** involves using data and analytical tools to measure and document progress toward goals.
- **Directing** requires coaching; delegating; and otherwise providing instruction to, taking charge of, and motivating supervisees as well as moving projects or plans toward their goals.
- **Staffing** means selecting and training people for specific job functions and giving them the associated responsibilities.

Some key "truths" that I and other supervisors have discovered:

- Supervising is not as easy as it looks when you're a staff member.
- Multitasking is a difficult but invaluable skill.
- Learn to set priorities.
- Rules and policies are helpful, but make sure to enforce them with compassion, empathy, and tact.
- The performance of your department or division (whether good or bad) is ultimately your responsibility, so avoid blaming others, such as your predecessors or supervisees, for failures or poor outcomes.
- On a supervisory team, communicate with your colleagues to avoid inconsistencies in supervision, such as only one supervisor handing out warnings when employees come in late—a discrepancy supervisees will quickly identify.
- In health care, almost every decision should boil down to how patient care is affected.
- You will encounter problems, no matter how competent or skilled at supervising you are.
- Don't hire someone just to fill a vacancy—find the right person for the job.
- Be present and accessible to your staff and know what's going on in your department or division.
- Don't hold your supervisees to any expectations you don't hold for yourself.

Precepting

Many resources exist to help those interested in becoming preceptors or teaching others. Contact the schools of pharmacy where you'd like to precept and ask about prerequisite training or education. Most schools offer packets of information to help you get your rotations up and running and develop basic precepting skills. Depending on the size of your employer and the amount of resources available at your institution, you may even have access to some site-specific materials or training tools. Some basic tips for precepting:

- **Plan ahead.** Establish goals, objectives, and schedules well before your student arrives on rotation.

- **Get organized.** Set aside resources and space for students to work. Organize your calendar to allocate time for mid-point and final evaluations, orientation at the beginning of the rotation, and one-on-one student activities you've identified.

- **Set clear expectations.** Make sure your students know where to be, when to be there, and exactly what is expected of them from the first day of the rotation. On the first day, I go over the evaluation tool to ensure they understand the criteria on which they will be assessed, and I give them a notebook that includes a schedule, list of goals and objectives for the rotation, and other important information.

— **Provide timely, specific feedback.** This includes mid-point and final evaluations as well as periodic feedback on activities, projects, and exercises. The more specific you can be, the better. For example, "Great job using the three prime questions to counsel that patient on her new inhaler" is better than "Great work counseling that patient." "I'd suggest you use more open-ended questions when verifying a patient's understanding" is better than "You should work to improve your patient counseling skills."

— **Teach your profession, not just your job.** I require my students to attend most, if not all, of my professional activities during the month they are on rotation with me. If I give a presentation out of town, they go with me. When I volunteer at the free clinic after work, or attend an early morning meeting before my shift begins, they come too. Show students all aspects of your life as a pharmacist, not just things you do on your regular paid shift.

Teaching

No matter where you are in your schooling or career, you probably have at least some experience presenting or teaching pharmacy-related information. Build on this and seek specific guidance on aspects of teaching you need to learn more about, such as developing objectives, creating a didactic lecture, establishing learning objectives, or public speaking.

In addition to the resources listed in Box 8-3 on page 141, you can get information from your employer, your local college, or in your community—such as public-speaking training with Toastmasters International (www.Toastmasters.org), a nonprofit that holds meetings in most cities and towns.

Tailor your teaching style to the needs and characteristics of your learner. Table 8-2 on page 139 draws upon the Myers-Briggs Type Indicator classifications discussed in Chapters 3 and 7 to give examples of how people with different characteristics may learn differently. Your MBTI type will also help you understand how you prefer to teach.

Below are tips to enhance your teaching skills for students of all learning styles.

— **Be enthusiastic.** If *you're* not excited about the topic you're teaching, how can you expect learners to be? If you have to teach a subject that's not of particular interest to you, at least find an unusual way to present the information or gauge understanding to keep your students' interest piqued.

— **Focus on mastery before grades.** Remind students that grasping the material is their most important goal. On the introductory hospital rotation I teach, I want students to leave with a basic understanding of how the hospital pharmacy operates, how the medication use process works, and how the pharmacy department fits into the overall scheme of things. As long as my students behave professionally and work toward this understanding, I assure them, they will do fine. I'd rather teach a C student who really works at absorbing information than an A student who regurgitates material to perform well on exams.

— **Require reflection.** As I noted in Chapter 3, I never liked writing "reflection statements," but now that I'm in practice, I'm so thankful I learned this skill. Contemplation allows me to think things through more thoroughly, understand myself and my priorities better, and set goals and objectives for the future. I ask the same of students, on a smaller scale, so they think about how each educational activity fits into their specific professional development plan and how they will use the new information.

— **Use a variety of techniques.** Even when I teach a didactic lecture, I try to incorporate a "show of hands" interaction, ask questions, and engage the audience. Many larger teaching facilities have audience response systems that allow you to carry out real-time polls to learn opinions, assess knowledge, or assure that learning objectives have been met. Students push a button on their response device to indicate their reply; results are immediately tabulated and shown on a screen. In smaller groups, you can incorporate small group discussions and tabletop exercises—theoretical situations, cases, or problems that a small group must respond to or solve. Using a combination of styles allows you to reach many different types of learners.

— **Encourage participation.** Research suggests that students who are more actively engaged with the material are more likely to retain the information. You can't *require* participation in all cases, but you can encourage and reward it. When I'm teaching a particular continuing education course for local pharmacists, I ask attendees to raise their hands if they need clarification, I ask questions to gauge the participants' understanding, and I provide a small chocolate candy to anyone who answers. (Chocolate is a big incentive to participate in *my* world!)

— **Explain why material is important.** Most difficult to learn is material that doesn't fit into the "big picture" just yet. Explain how what you're teaching is important, fits a larger learning plan, or relates to the learners' personal or professional goals. Information is easier for learners to retain if they have a purpose in mind for its future use.

— **Use a little humor.** Teaching doesn't have to be all business. Add touches of humor to engage students and help them retain material. When I teach a course in basic Spanish for pharmacists, I interject stories about humorous results from misinterpretations—such as that the car made by Chevrolet called the Nova didn't sell well in Spanish-speaking countries because "no va" means "doesn't go." Humor can break down barriers between you and your students and help everyone relax.

Table 8-2

Characteristics of Learners by MBTI Type

Extroverted Learners	Introverted Learners
– Need action and interaction to learn – Enjoy discussions to find solutions – Value frequent feedback – Require shorter "think time" – Need breaks to talk or move, to gain energy for silent reading and writing activities	– Learn best when they have time for reflection – Require longer "think time" – Prefer to ask and discuss one question or issue at a time – Favor silent reading and writing activities
Sensing Learners	**Intuitive Learners**
– Like to start with factual information before moving to broader concepts – Like step-by-step processes, policies, details, rules, and proportional logic – Ask questions immediately to clarify assignments – Do not want to waste time doing anything wrong	– Find step-by-step processes, details, rules, and proportional logic frustrating – Think "out-of-the-box" – Use imagination – Question basic assumptions – Ask their questions five minutes after receiving directions – Are sometimes misperceived as poor listeners
Thinking Learners	**Feeling Learners**
– Look for logical explanations, cause-effect or if-then arguments, and universal rules or truths – Seem to enjoy arguments – Strive to be objective – Appeal to sense of equality and fairness	– Consider the impact a decision might have on the people involved – Have trouble functioning where putdowns and other forms of disharmony are common – Need specific praise in their critiques – Appreciate the contributions of others – Seek to understand the opinions of others

continued on page 140

Table 8-2

continued

Judging Learners	Perceiving Learners
— Seem to have built-in clocks: are able to plan out their work and work their plan — Often start working on assignments as soon as they receive them — Seem to be able to estimate how long a project will take them — Feel stressed in ways that inhibit both their creativity and their accuracy if they have to wait until the last minute — May not gather enough information or consider alternative ways to complete a project — Are on time and prepared — Want conclusions and closure — Are organized and don't like to waste time	— Live more in the moment, taking a spontaneous approach to life — May seem lazy, late, or irresponsible — Like options and appreciate opportunities to discuss them — Understand that being flexible opens opportunities — Are better at staying open to new ideas and considering alternate ways to approach an assignment or task — Do their best work under pressure — Often underestimate how long a project will take — Need different time management tools, such as planning backward and building interim goals for larger projects

Adapted from:

1. Missouri Nurse Preceptor Academy. Tips for types: MBTI preferences. *Preceptor News.* August 2008.

2. Missouri Nurse Preceptor Academy. Put your MBTI personality type to "work" for you. *Preceptor News.* August 2008.

Box 8-3

Additional Resources to Help You Hone Skills

Ambulatory Care

ACCP Ambulatory Care New Practitioner Survival Guide/Resource Manual
(Blair MM. Lenexa, Kan: American College of Clinical Pharmacy; 2008.)
Both new and seasoned ambulatory care clinicians can learn from these detailed examples of successful clinical practices and lists of references for further study.

Business and Finance

Financial Management for Health-System Pharmacists
(Wilson AI, ed. Bethesda, Md: American Society of Health-System Pharmacists; 2008.)
Learn the basics of finance and accounting for institutional health care and take advantage of fundamental financial management tools that relate not only to the pharmacy department, but the hospital and health care system. Topics include principles of accounting and budgeting, forecasting pharmaceutical expenditures, cost management, and controlling operating results.

How to Develop a Business Plan for Pharmacy Services
(Schumock GT, Stubbings J. 2nd ed. Lenexa, Kan: American College of Clinical Pharmacy; 2007.)
This book helps you plan, develop, launch, and evaluate business services in the pharmacy field using a systematic approach. A step-by-step analysis and insightful questions lead you through business plan development; you also get sample business plans and a companion CD-ROM.

Understanding Pharmacy Reimbursement
(Vogenberg FR, ed. Bethesda, Md: American Society of Health-System Pharmacists; 2005.)
This comprehensive guide examines current issues, strategies, requirements, risk management, consumer awareness, and the evolution of pharmacy reimbursement. It includes practical instruction for a variety of practice settings, including hospitals, home care, long-term care, community, and retail.

continued on page 142

Box 8-3

continued

Collaborative and Patient-Centered Practice

Building a Successful Collaborative Pharmacy Practice: Guidelines and Tools
(Bennett M, Wedret JJ, eds. Washington, D.C.: American Pharmacists Association; 2004.)
This book is full of guidelines, tips, and ready-to-use forms to help you establish collaborative practice arrangements, consult with teams of practitioners, re-engineer your workflow, manage and market your practice, and obtain reimbursement for services. It also includes tools to help you monitor drug regimens, report patient care, and advise patients about proper medication use and health habits. It includes a CD-ROM so you can adapt documents for your own practice.

Collaborative Drug Therapy Management Handbook
(Tracy SA, Clegg CA, eds. Bethesda, Md: American Society of Health-System Pharmacists; 2007.)
Designed as a starting point for establishing a collaborative practice, this book addresses the core elements necessary, includes in-depth sample guidelines, and presents case studies illustrating how to use the guidelines. Chapters also cover credentialing and measuring outcomes.

Managing the Patient-Centered Pharmacy
(Hagel HP, Rovers JP, eds. Washington, D.C.: American Pharmaceutical Association; 2002.)
This is the first book examining the management decisions and processes needed to successfully implement a pharmaceutical care practice in both community and hospital pharmacies. The chapters, written by experienced academicians and practitioners, cover changing to a patient care-oriented practice model, use of automation, staff motivation, creating a business plan, and financial management.

Developing Management Skills

ASHP's Management Pearls
(Ash D, ed. Bethesda, Md: American Society of Health-System Pharmacists; 2008.)
This volume illustrates creative ways to approach issues and solve problems and includes examples of tools, techniques, and interventions that have improved pharmacy management in both U.S. and foreign health systems.

continued on page 143

Box 8-3

continued

Managing & Leading: 44 Lessons Learned for Pharmacists
(Bush P, Walesh SG. Bethesda, Md: American Society of Health-System Pharmacists; 2008.)
These useful ideas and tools for pharmacists, residents, and students help you improve your skills and more effectively approach the non-technical aspects of working with colleagues, administrators, vendors, clients, and patients. Each lesson contains a key idea and practical suggestions for applying it.

Pharmacy Management: Essentials for All Practice Settings
(Desselle SP, Zgarrick DP. 2nd cd. New York: McGraw-Hill Medical; 2008.)
From operations management and purchasing to Medicare Part D, this guide examines vital pharmacy management topics across all practice settings. It's packed with advice from top experts who take you through principles applicable to all aspects of pharmacy practice, from managing money to managing stress.

Staff Development for Pharmacy Practice
(Nimmo CM, ed. Bethesda, Md: American Society of Health-System Pharmacists; 2000.)
This easy-to-use manual provides a systematic approach to developing pharmacy staff skills for direct patient care. Grounded in the principles of instructional systems design, it covers forming clear expectations of training outcomes, linking methods of instruction to desired performance, and accurately assessing skills learned.

Supervision: A Pharmacy Perspective
(Wick JY. Washington, D.C.: American Pharmacists Association; 2003.)
Incorporating the pharmacy perspective in every discussion, this book covers motivating employees, bringing about change, workplace rules and expectations, communication, productive meetings, rewards and discipline, handling complaints and grievances, U.S. Labor laws, licensure, credentialing, malpractice, documentation, and peer review.

Medication Therapy Management (MTM)

100 MTM Tips for the Pharmacist
(Millonig MK. Washington, D.C.: American Pharmacists Association; 2008.)
These tips from many settings help pharmacists who are struggling to integrate patient care and medication therapy management in their practices. It's an easy-to-use source of new ideas, from getting started to advocacy to educating others.

continued on page 144

Box 8-3

continued

Medication Therapy Management Services: A Critical Review
(The Lewin Group. Available at: www.lewin.com/content/publications/3179.pdf.)
The American Pharmacists Association commissioned The Lewin Group to identify existing MTM services standards of practice and develop an illustrative model for payers. The resulting report is a great resource for those designing MTM programs under the Medicare Modernization Act of 2003 or expanding MTM services in both the public and private sectors.

The Pharmacist's Guide to Compensation for Medication Therapy Management Services
(Hogue MD, Bluml BM, eds. Washington, D.C.: American Pharmacists Association; 2008.)
Inside you'll find timely information about compensation for providing MTM services in major practice settings as well as practical information on documentation and billing, resource materials, and sample forms.

Precepting

Preceptor Training and Resource Network
(Pharmacist's Letter. Available at: http://pharmacistsletter.therapeuticresearch.com; click the "Preceptor Home" link in the navigation.)
The Preceptor Training and Resource Network provides a platform to easily connect pharmacists with teaching resources and preceptor training programs and to enhance their precepting skills. You get sample assignments and projects, evaluation tools, and orientation checklists and can participate in live webinars on effective precepting by pharmacy faculty. You can also receive continuing education credits.

Preceptor's Handbook for Pharmacists
(Cuellar L, Ginsburg D. 2nd ed. Bethesda, Md: American Society of Health-System Pharmacists; 2009.)
A trusted reference, this book contains practical advice on the various aspects of precepting and covers necessary skills, mentoring, experiential teaching, law and ethics, and professionalism, among other topics.

continued on page 145

Box 8-3

continued

Preceptors' Perspectives on Benefits of Precepting Student Pharmacists to Students, Preceptors, and the Profession

(Skrabal MZ, Kahaleh AA, Nemire RE, et al. *J Am Pharm Assoc.* 2006;46(5):605-12.) This article describes the shortage of and need for pharmacy preceptors, the benefits of precepting, and the qualities of successful preceptors. The authors also offer the results of their literature evaluation on the subject of pharmacy precepting, guidance on becoming a successful preceptor, and advice from three pharmacists who have won preceptor of the year awards.

Public Relations and Marketing

Marketing for Pharmacists

(Holdford DA. 2nd ed. Washington, D.C.: American Pharmacists Association; 2007.) As this book makes clear, pharmacists in all settings can use marketing techniques to build their practices, develop innovative services, and generate business for their employers or organizations. You learn how to develop a marketing plan, apply marketing strategies to pharmacy problems, and improve your ability to attract and retain patients and customers.

Public Relations for Pharmacists

(Pugliese TL. 2nd ed. Washington, D.C.: American Pharmacists Association; 2008.) The only book on public relations designed for pharmacy provides you with tools to advance your practice and the profession through public relations, media relations, community involvement, and special events. In addition to providing guidance for working with the media and writing materials such as news releases and blogs, the book gives sample messages and lists of do's and don'ts.

Maintaining Your Personal Life

When your career is in full swing, it can feel as if your personal and professional lives are in a tug-of-war. Seems like it should be easy to keep up with what you love—friends, family, hobbies—but work can take over, if you let it.

Managing your money can be tough, too. When you're getting a regular paycheck, it's tempting to think that's all you need—the rest will take care of itself. But along with earning money comes the responsibility of managing it and planning ahead for later stages of life.

Work–Life Balance

In the article "Work Life Balance: Tips and Techniques" in the Careers section of About.com, career coach Thomas J. Denham points out these signs that work–life balance has run amuck:
– Merely trying to get through the day.
– Barely making it to the end of the week and feeling completely exhausted when you get home.
– Feeling that life is a merry-go-round and you want to get off.
– Having a constant sense of falling behind and never catching up in life.

At some point, everyone with a career feels out of balance. And not everyone's idea of a well-balanced life is the same. You have to find the mix that works for you and allows you to achieve both your personal and professional goals. Over time, the best balance for you may change. I am still learning how to maintain balance—it's not easy—and have found excellent tips and helpful readings. Some basics:

— **Don't feel guilty.** While you're at home, why waste time worrying about the things you should be getting done for work? The reverse is true, too—at work, don't worry about things piling up at home. It won't improve an imbalanced work–life situation to beat yourself up about it.

— **Prioritize.** Determine what is most important to you in your life and list these priorities. Make sure your list reflects how you *truly* feel rather than how you *think* you should feel. Some experts argue that having a concrete idea of your top priorities allows you to maintain a better balance.

— **Don't take it home with you.** You shouldn't take work home unless it's absolutely unavoidable. Be in the moment no matter where you are—and if you're home, concentrate on your personal life. If you must work at home, schedule specific times to get the work done and don't let the hours overtake all your personal time. I keep a notepad by my bed and another in my living room so I can jot anything I forgot to follow up on that day at work. This way, I get "to-do" items out of my thoughts until I'm back at work.

— **Learn how to say no.** This skill empowers you to spend time on what's most important to you based on the priorities you've established. As a card-carrying "people-pleaser," I've struggled and felt guilty about declining tasks, but I've learned that saying no gives me the opportunity to become excellent at selected things rather than average at many. The more you practice saying no, the easier it gets. Say it in a firm, polite, and professional way and phrase it simply; you don't need to apologize or explain. For example:
  - "I'd love to help but I'm already overextended."
  - "That doesn't work for me."
  - "I prefer not to."
  - "I'm not able to do that."

— **Get organized.** Scheduling and organizing can improve your work–life balance because it helps you make the best use of your time.

— **Schedule time for exercise, sleep, relaxation, and enjoyment.** These are the first things to go when your work–life balance starts to shift. Build them into your calendar and remember that an adequate amount of each allows you to function better at home and at work.

— **Delegate at home and at work.** Ask teammates or colleagues to help with tasks at work, and delegate when you can. You'll never be able to do it all, no matter what your expertise is or in what setting you practice. Likewise, rely on others in your household or personal life to lighten your load and make sure everything gets done.

- **Embrace technology.** Technology can be a wonderful time-saver when you use it to get organized. Use a smartphone or personal digital assistant to maintain your calendar, keep you on schedule, and put prioritized "to do" lists at your fingertips for both work and home.

- **Don't let technology overrun you.** The flip side is that technology can take up all the time it saves you. Turn off the BlackBerry, iPhone, cell phone, or pager during personal activities so you can fully connect with the important people in your life.

- **If you get overwhelmed, speak up.** It's perfectly acceptable to tell your boss you're feeling overextended at work or to tell friends and family that personal obligations are overwhelming you. When important people in your life know how you're feeling, they can help you get things back in balance and they are less likely to be disappointed or upset if you can't meet their expectations.

Box 9-1, Selected Reading on Life Balance and Stress Management, lists books that offer detailed tips, guidance, assessments, and strategies for keeping your life in balance and stress under control.

Box 9-1

Selected Reading on Life Balance and Stress Management

CEO Dad: How to Avoid Getting Fired by Your Family
(Stern T. Mountain View, Calif: Davies-Black Publishing; 2007.)
Packed with insightful cartoons, this book takes a lighthearted yet realistic look at the conflicts between business executives and the people they love. Inspired by his own journey of a being a CEO who drove his family over the edge, the author talks about alienating employees and potential clients, treating his children like business protégés, and ultimately, being humiliated by his family on reality TV.

Don't Sweat the Small Stuff—and It's All Small Stuff
(Carlson R. New York: Hyperion; 1997.)
This popular and cheerful book offers 100 meditations designed to help you appreciate being alive, keep your emotions in perspective, and cherish other people.

Get a Grip! Overcoming Stress and Thriving in the Workplace
(Losyk B. Hoboken, N.J.: John Wiley & Sons; 2005.)
Get practical tips and simple exercises for relieving everyday stress in this book, geared toward workers based in the office or at home. Learn techniques to relax your mind, body, and spirit, get to the heart of your stress, and find effective ways to cope.

continued on page 150

Box 9-1

continued

Harvard Business Review on Work and Life Balance
(Harvard Business Review. Boston: Harvard Business School Press; 2000.)
Fundamental information to help you stay competitive in a fast-moving world is covered in articles ranging from an in-depth look at the "mommy-track" to perspectives on telecommuting. It's a great book to help professionals grasp the delicate balance between professional and personal life.

Life Is Not Work, Work Is Not Life: Simple Reminders for Finding Balance in a 24/7 World
(Johnston RK, Smith JW. Berkeley, Calif: Wilcat Canyon Press; 2001.)
This book by a theologian and a market researcher contains brief essays combining their own wisdom and the latest market research to address the modern problem of working more and enjoying life less. After a 20th century defined by work, including industrialization, downsizing, working couples, daycare, second careers, and 24/7, the 21st century brings a deep-seated need to balance a strong work ethic with leisure-time enjoyment.

Life Matters: Creating Dynamic Balance of Work, Family, Time, and Money
(Merrill AR. New York: McGraw-Hill; 2003.)
Written by efficiency experts, this book guides you in exploring your priorities and expanding your capacity for happiness and fulfillment. It includes a self-assessment quiz to evaluate the vital life elements of work, family, time, and money and helps you examine the gap between what you value and your daily life. Also covered are using technology to create more time and the concept of "dynamic investing," which includes intangibles such as energy, relationships, and integrity.

The Relaxation & Stress Reduction Workbook
(Davis M, Eshelman ER, McKay M, et al. 6th ed. Oakland, Calif: New Harbinger Publications; 2008.)
Full of self-assessment tools and calming techniques, this hefty workbook helps promote physical and emotional well-being in chapters on relaxation, thought stopping, body awareness, goal setting, time management, assertiveness training, and other topics. First introduced in 1980, the book received praise for presenting a comprehensive look at stress, its physical manifestations, and the many ways it can be managed.

continued on page 151

Box 9-1

continued

Stop Living Your Job, Start Living Your Life: 85 Simple Strategies to Achieve Work/Life Balance
(Molloy A. Berkeley, Calif: Ulysses Press; 2005.)
Remaking your life to match your personal priorities is the focus of this book, which is packed with interactive tools, quizzes, and tips to help you control your responsibilities rather than letting them control you. Practical advice covers everything from decluttering space and managing finances to staying committed and pursuing dreams.

The Stress Management Handbook
(Leyden-Rubenstein L. New Canaan, Conn: Keats Publishing; 1999.)
This easy-to-read book combines scientific background, compelling success stories, and comprehensive approaches to stress management. Learn more than 50 practical strategies for physical relaxation; overcoming stressful thoughts, beliefs, and emotions; getting needs met; self-reflection; communication skills; self-acceptance; listening to your inner voice; and many other topics.

Stress Reduction for Busy People: Finding Peace in an Anxious World
(Groves D. Novato, Calif: New World Library; 2004.)
Some simple choices can change bad habits into good ones and give you a few minutes each day to take care of your body, mind, and soul, the author posits. She presents helpful techniques such as "reframing" and "facts not stories" for healthier emotional responses, and she provides other practical tips.

Striking a Balance: Work, Family, Life
(Drago RW. Boston: Dollars & Sense; 2007.)
In this book, an economist and work-life expert unmasks the real reasons most Americans lead unbalanced lives. He taps a vast body of research and new findings from his own studies to examine deeply-held beliefs that lead to out-of-balance lives. His final chapter provides a road map for change—so as to improve your life balance, income inequality, and the "new gender gap" of women who care for others.

Nontraditional Work Arrangements

One way to achieve work–life balance may be to look for nontraditional work arrangements, such as those described below. Consider asking about these options when inquiring about jobs or while on interviews. Each comes with a unique set of challenges and its own pros and cons. Be sure that the arrangement will not hold you back from your professional goals and that it helps you achieve what's most important to you in your life.

Family-Friendly Employment

A family-friendly policy is any approach or benefit designed to help employees achieve a satisfactory work–life balance. Although such policies are often introduced to make it easier for mothers to work, legally they have to be open to all employees. Such policies may involve flexible hours, time spent working from home, child care or elder care provisions, or paid time off for participating in community activities or volunteer work. Benefits to the employer include better employee retention, higher motivation, and increased job satisfaction.

Job Sharing

In this scenario, two people share the responsibilities of one full-time position, which can work well for both employees and employers. Two pharmacists who work for me share a job; one is a new mother and the other left retirement to maintain his community pharmacy skills. Neither desires a full-time job, but both want to stay in the workforce. One works three days per week and the other works two. Scheduling for job-sharers can actually be easier than scheduling full-time employees. I can be more flexible in accommodating their requests for time off because the two pharmacists who share the job can fill in for each other or trade shifts.

Job sharing can involve more effort on your part to keep everyone on the same page about projects and activities and to make sure they know exactly when you will and won't be at work. You may need to let others contact you when you're off duty if there's an emergency or they need information. Have a written plan for divvying responsibilities so that you, your boss, and the other job-sharer are clear about which items are your responsibility and which are not.

Telecommuting

Telecommuting is working from home for a business and communicating via personal computer, the Internet, telephone, and communications software. In some telecommuting positions you work from home regularly and spend very little time at the physical worksite, while others involve working from home one or more days a week and going to the worksite the other days. Benefits include increased flexibility in your schedule, less time spent commuting, and improved productivity by avoiding the distractions and hectic atmosphere at the worksite. Employers may be able to spend less money on overhead, including utilities and supplies, when employees telecommute.

On the down side, telecommuting can isolate you from others at work: teammates, colleagues, supervisors, other health care professionals, and patients. It's harder to build relationships and stay in the forefront of people's minds for projects when you're not physically present. Telecommuting may also require more "accountability" than when you're at the worksite each day, in the form of scheduled calls, progress updates, and activity reports. For some people, telecommuting can make it harder to balance work and personal life because both take place in the same physical location.

Stress Management

If you're exhibiting signs of stress, your first step is to identify the stressor. It sounds easy, but the true source of your stress may not be as obvious as you think. A helpful approach is to keep a "stress journal." Each time you feel anxious, overwhelmed, or irritated, write an entry that notes:
– What caused your stress
– How you felt, both physically and emotionally
– How you acted in response
– What you did to make yourself feel better

After writing this information down, you'll start to see a pattern that sheds light on your stressors. Next, look at how you deal with them. If you tend to resort to any of the unhealthy approaches below, you'll harm yourself in the long run.
– Smoking
– Drinking too much
– Overeating or undereating
– Zoning out for hours in front of the TV or computer
– Withdrawing from friends, family, and activities
– Using pills or drugs to relax
– Sleeping too much
– Procrastinating
– Filling up every minute of the day to avoid facing problems
– Taking out your stress on others (lashing out, angry outbursts, physical violence)

Healthy ways to deal with stress fall into four categories:
1. Avoid the stressor
2. Alter the stressor
3. Adapt to the stressor
4. Accept the stressor

Table 9-1 gives examples of steps you can take in each category to cope with stress. Often a combination of approaches helps the most. You can also reduce stress by maintaining your work–life balance, learning relaxation techniques, and establishing a healthy lifestyle.

Table 9-1

Coping with Stress

Avoid	Alter	Adapt	Accept
Learn to say "no" Prioritize (Distinguish between "must do" and "should do"). Avoid particularly stressful situations (such as traffic jams) by finding an alternative (taking a longer, less congested route).	Communicate with others if you are feeling stressed about something. Sharing may present a mutual solution to a stressful situation. Ask someone to change his or her behavior, and be willing to do the same in return. Improve your time management skills to avoid running behind and being ill prepared.	Focus on the positive. Set reasonable expectations of yourself. Setting goals that you can't achieve can make you stressed and set you up to fail. Reframe problems. Looking at things from a different angle can help make them less stressful.	Don't try to control the uncontrollable. Share your feelings with others such as a friend, family member, or counselor, which helps you release pent-up stress and can be cathartic.
Adapted from: www.helpguide.org			

Exercising regularly, eating a healthy diet, reducing caffeine and sugar, avoiding alcohol or drinking in moderation, avoiding cigarettes and drugs, and getting enough sleep can really increase your resistance to stress. It also helps to learn formal relaxation techniques, such as meditation, or to allow time for other healthy ways to relax such as:

- Reading
- Spending time outdoors
- Catching up with a friend
- Exercising
- Writing
- Taking a long bath
- Lighting scented candles
- Savoring a warm cup of coffee or tea
- Playing with a pet
- Getting a massage
- Listening to soothing music

Think of these healthy and relaxing practices as "required" for a successful life. If you skip them, you'll pay. I say this from experience. I truly am a workaholic. I would often pride myself on working harder and longer hours than others. I thought that the more things I checked off my to-do list by putting in more time, the less stressed I'd be. But the opposite was true. Stress affected my personal life, my happiness and well-being, and even my health.

At one point several years ago, I was pulling long hours, not exercising, and eating poorly because I told myself "I don't have time." Soon I found out from my physician that my cholesterol was high and I was overweight. (She didn't need to tell me about the weight, though—I knew because none of my clothes fit.) I was irritable and no fun to be around, although I didn't notice at the time. The day I bent over in the pharmacy and split a pair of scrub pants down the middle was the last straw. I *had* to do something.

I'd played soccer and field hockey in school and I certainly knew how important diet and exercise are, but I'd let work take priority over my wellness for too long. I joined Weight Watchers and started back at the gym. Now I'm down more than 30 pounds, my cholesterol is normal, my clothes fit again, and I *feel* so much better. Following a healthy routine makes it easier for me to cope with the work and personal stresses that come along every day.

Financial Planning

Of course, the hugely important topic of financial planning can't be thoroughly covered in this brief section, so to give you the basics, I've adapted tips from an excellent presentation by pharmacist C. Barry Hiatt, staff development coordinator at North Carolina Baptist Hospital in Winston-Salem. You can view the presentation at the North Carolina Association of Pharmacists' website at www.ncpharmacists.org; in the menu to the left, click Pharmacists, and in the drop-down menu that appears, click New Practitioner Network to locate the presentation. Hiatt points out that you must:

- Create and maintain a budget to keep your spending under control.
- Avoid debt.
  - If you have debts (credit cards, consumer loans, or others) pay them off.
  - Start with the lowest balance and work up to the largest.
  - A reasonable goal is to become debt-free, other than the mortgage on your house.
- Live on less than you earn.
- Have a financial plan and reassess it periodically.
  - See the brochures *Nervous? Time to Reassess (or Make) a Financial Plan* and *Thinking the Unthinkable: What Everyone Needs to Know About Estate Planning* in the American Pharmacists Association (APhA) Financial Planning Resource Center at www.pharmacist.com. The resource center is described in Box 9-2.
- Determine if and when you need assistance with financial planning and investing.
  - See the brochure *Cutting Through the Confusion: Where to Turn for Help with Your Investments* in the Financial Planning Resource Center at www.pharmacist.com.

Box 9-2

The Financial Planning Resource Center

The American Pharmacists Association (APhA) and the Financial Planning Association (FPA) have joined forces to help new practitioners better manage their money and discover the value of financial planning. Go to www.pharmacist.com, click on New Practitioners, and you'll find the link for Financial Planning Resource Center. Among the benefits of this collaboration:

- Access to PlannerSearch (exclusively for APhA members), which allows you to search for professionals who are certified financial planners (CFP) by city and state, zip code, radius, last name, and even specialty. You can search for financial planners who offer free initial consultations and access the FPA's "Ask a CFP Professional" email hotline to ask general financial planning questions and receive answers from CFP professionals.
- Financial Planning Strategies Workshops offered at many APhA Annual Meetings.
- FPA's Financial Planning Perspectives articles in *Transitions*, the quarterly newsletter published for members of the APhA New Practitioner Network. Back issues are available online at www.pharmacist.com on the New Practitioners page.
- Financial planning brochures available at www.pharmacist.com on topics ranging from buying a home to investing, financial planning, and estate planning.

When I said basics, I meant basics, so let's quickly review the purposes of money—summarized in Table 9-2. Based on the information in this table, the tips below are categorized according to the purpose for which you will be using the funds.

Table 9-2

The Purposes of Money

Spending	Food Clothes Housing Transportation Vacations College Educations
Saving	Emergency Fund Investments Retirement
Giving	Local Church Charities Gifts Endowments

Adapted from: Hiatt CB. *Financial Planning for Pharmacy Residents*. Available at: www.ncpharmacists.org/displaycommon.cfm?an=1&subarticlenbr=66.

Spending

For most of us, spending money is much more fun than earning it. But allowing your spending to get out of control can turn your life upside down. The key is to spend your money wisely (which is helped greatly by developing a budget) and avoid spending more than you earn.

Tips for Buying a Home

Buying one's own home has long been the American dream—a dream that has been challenged by the mortgage crisis of the early 21st century. Keep the following in mind:
- You can't really afford all of the mortgage amount you'll qualify for.
- Save until you have at least 20% of the purchase price for a down payment.
- Your mortgage payment should not exceed 25% of your take-home pay.
- See the brochure *Financial Planning for a Home of Your Own* in the Financial Planning Resource Center at www.pharmacist.com.

Saving

Everyone's savings goals are different, depending on their situation and stage in life. To save effectively, you must know what you want to accomplish with your money, such as buying a home, launching a business, educating your children, or retiring by the age of 60. Think through what's most important to you; then set and prioritize your financial goals so you achieve what you want.

Tips for Starting an Emergency Fund

You never know what the future holds. One of the smartest things you can do as soon as you start your career is to build a cash reserve to draw on when the unexpected happens.

- Initially shoot for $2000.
- Gradually build up to the goal of three to six months of living expenses.
- Keep your emergency reserve fully funded and protected.

Tips for Investing

Investing is a huge topic and I can't even scratch the surface, other than giving you a few rules of thumb.

- Invest 15% of your gross income annually. You will need to start slowly, but start now.
- Each of your financial goals will demand a different strategy and investment vehicle, depending on its type. See Table 9-3 for a summary of goals, time frames, and associated investment vehicles.
- Individual stocks are typically too risky for the new investor.
- Roth IRAs (individual retirement accounts) are a must while you can qualify; those eligible must fall under a certain income cap, which is different depending on whether you are single or married. (These caps change, so check each year to see if you qualify.)
- Choose mutual funds for your 401(k) or 403(b). (See Table 9-4 for definitions of these plans.) Morningstar (www.morningstar.com) is an example of a good place to start learning about mutual funds.
- Consult a professional investment adviser. Look at the person's track record for the past 5- and 10-year periods by checking the Central Registration Depository (CRD) and the Investment Adviser Public Disclosure (IAPD), found on the website of the U.S. Securities and Exchange Commission (www.sec.gov), or simply ask the adviser for this information. Find detailed information in the article, *Protect Your Money: Check Out Brokers and Investment Advisers*, also at www.sec.gov.
- See the brochure *20 Keys to Being a Smarter Investor* in the Financial Planning Resource Center at www.pharmacist.com.

Table 9-3

Investment Time Frames, Goals, and Vehicles

Time Frame	Goals	Investment Vehicle
Short-term (1–3 years)	Down payment on home New car Vacation	Money market account Certificates of deposit
Intermediate-term (3–10 years)	Children's education Trade up to a larger home Start a business Change careers	Education IRA Individual stocks and bonds Stock mutual funds Balanced mutual funds
Long-term (10 years or more)	Retirement Vacation home World cruise	401(k) IRA Roth IRA Variable annuities Growth mutual funds

Adapted from Hiatt CB. *Financial Planning for Pharmacy Residents*. Available at: www.ncpharmacists.org/displaycommon.cfm?an=1&subarticlenbr=66.

Tips for Retirement Planning

You have to start investing now for your retirement, even though retirement feels far away.

- The best step you can take in investing for retirement is to maximize your employer's 401(k) or 403(b) plan. (See Table 9-4 for definitions and descriptions of common retirement planning options.)
- Set aside at least what your employer matches in a retirement plan. It's "free money," and not only do you save for retirement, but you also reduce your taxable income.
- If you're already employed, contact your company's human resources department for more information on your retirement plan.

Tips for Insurance

Sorting through insurance plans and the types of coverage they provide is challenging. Still, it's time well spent, because having the proper insurance can make all the difference when disaster strikes. Be sure to get the right amount of coverage from companies that have good track records for paying claims and satisfying customers.

- The insurance you should buy depends on where you are in life and your personal and family needs.

Table 9-4

Some Retirement Planning Options

Type of Plan	Description
Individual Retirement Account (IRAs and Roth IRAs)	IRAs and Roth IRAs are widely recommended for workers with no company-sponsored retirement plan. Most account holders can invest an annual maximum of $2000 in an IRA. Traditional IRAs are the most popular choice among investors because of their up-front tax deduction on contributions. There are no tax deductions on Roth IRA contributions, but withdrawals are tax-free if the plan is held for five years and the account holder is over age $59\frac{1}{2}$. Roth IRAs are best for young savers whose money has a long time to grow tax-free.
401(k) or 403(b)	Investors love these tax-sheltered savings plans in part because of the matching contributions offered by many employers. Participants can put in up to 15% of their annual salary. A 401(k) plan cannot require more than one year of employment service for employees to be eligible to make their own contributions. These plans are portable and can be rolled over into an IRA or another 401(k) when an employee changes jobs. A 403(b) plan is similar to a 401(k) except it's for employees of educational institutions and certain other nonprofit organizations.
Pension Plan	Cash-balance pension plans, such as the 401(k), are quickly replacing the old company-paid defined-benefit pension plans, which usually require the worker to stay with the company for many years—often for 20 years or longer. In a defined-benefit pension plan, an employer commits to paying its employee a specific benefit for life beginning at his or her retirement. Today's job-hopping workers have pushed employers to install the cash-balance pension because they can take a lump-sum payout with them when they leave the company. The payout can be rolled over into an IRA or taken as cash. Few companies offer defined-benefit pension plans any longer.

continued on page 161

Table 9-4

continued

Employee Stock Ownership Plan (ESOP)	The National Center for Employee Ownership defines the ESOP as "a retirement-type plan in which a trust holds stock in the employee-participants' names; after they leave (whether due to quitting, retirement, etc.), they cash in on the proceeds due them."
	ESOPs may place too many eggs in one basket. If the stock does well, you might get rich. If the stock falls, your retirement fund may not be worth much. For more information, visit the National Center for Employee Ownership website at www.nceo.org.

Adapted from: Hiatt CB. *Financial Planning for Pharmacy Residents*. Available at: www.ncpharmacists.org/displaycommon.cfm?an=1&subarticlenbr=66.

- Only buy "term" life insurance.
- See the brochure *Choosing the Right Insurance for Your Life's Stages* in the Financial Planning Resource Center at www.pharmacist.com.

Giving

So much of life's satisfaction is about giving back. Part of your financial plan or annual budget should include donating funds.

- You decide how, when, and why to donate. You might give to your church, a charity, a pharmacy association or foundation, a school, or some other agency—either in one lump sum annually or smaller amounts throughout the year. For example, I donate to the foundation at the hospital where I work by way of monthly paycheck deductions. Choose a cause that's important to you. Decide your donation amount and schedule, and plan for it. If you think to yourself, "I'll do it later," it might never get done.
- No matter what your motivation, enjoy giving some money away. Helping the less fortunate is a great reason to give; you can also give to a charity that helped you in the past or give in honor of a loved one.
- Remember that donations to qualified organizations are tax deductible.

Maintaining Your Professional Life

"Get involved in pharmacy associations. Just being a member isn't enough. Volunteering and joining committees helps you develop a network and shape your future. I owe much of who I am today to my involvement with associations."

—Stephen M. Feldman, CEO of the ICPS Group and past president of the American Society of Consultant Pharmacists

In most pharmacy careers, as compared with other professions, the difference between the entry-level salary of a new graduate and the salary of a pharmacist who has spent many years in the profession is not great. Whether you see this lack of salary growth as good or bad, the reality is that entry-level salaries in pharmacy tend to be fairly substantial, allowing you to pay off school loans, start an emergency fund, and begin to enjoy some of your hard-earned cash more quickly than you might in some other careers.

The down side is that in most cases, financial incentives are not a huge motivator for pharmacists to take higher-ranking or more difficult positions. The amount of increase in salary a pharmacist might be offered to take a role such as "pharmacist-in-charge" is often not perceived as proportional to the amount of increased workload or stress. Of course, many reasons other than money can motivate you to keep learning and challenging yourself professionally. You may need to take a different approach to pursuing professional development than your colleagues in other professions, because career growth won't always happen naturally by climbing a ladder to higher positions in your organization. This chapter looks at ways to stay on track with your professional development now that getting an education is not your full-time job.

Keep on Top of Continuing Education

First and foremost, make sure you understand the continuing education (CE) requirements for every state in which you hold a pharmacy license. Don't wait until the last minute to discover you don't have enough education hours to renew your license at the end of the year. Otherwise, you'll probably have to quickly attend any education programs you can find, whether the subject matter interests you or not.

Plan ahead to attend programs and activities that meet your personal goals and professional interests. Also investigate nontraditional ways of obtaining CE hours in your state. For example, in North Carolina I can receive up to five live hours of CE credit for precepting students and up to five live hours for volunteering at a free clinic, and I can get credit for taking Spanish language classes to help me better communicate with my Spanish-speaking patients. I already do these three things anyway, and they all count toward my CE credits. Check your state board of pharmacy's website or call them to find out more about your own requirements.

Employ the Principle of Continuous Professional Development

Continuous Professional Development (CPD), a systematic and self-directed approach to professional learning, is an emerging model in the U.S. that has been studied and adopted in other countries, such as the United Kingdom and Canada. States studying the concept include North Carolina, Indiana, Iowa, Washington, and Wisconsin. Minutes from a meeting of the North Carolina Board of Pharmacy define CPD as "a self-directed, ongoing, systematic and outcome-focused approach to learning and professional development with five components: reflect, plan, act, evaluate, and record and review."

The goal of CPD programs is to allow individual pharmacists to structure their own educational plan so the objectives and outcomes are more relevant to their professional interests and practice site. Eventually, CPD programs might be how we obtain our CE credit to maintain licensure. Whether this happens or not, it's very helpful to follow the principles of CPD to maintain your professional practice, including:
- Developing a learning plan.
- Scheduling and planning learning activities that best fit your individual needs throughout the year.
- Incorporating professional learning into your regular activities.
- Keeping a record of ways your learning improved your performance and competence.

For more information on the continuous professional development concept, visit www.pharmacist.com, www.wsparx.org, or www.ncpharmacists.org and search for "CPD."

Update Your Portfolio and Curriculum Vitae

When your pharmacy school or residency program required you to prepare a curriculum vitae and professional portfolio, you may have been like me; you waited until the last minute to pull together all your presentations, projects, and other items. Maybe you had the same thought I did: "This would have been so much easier if I'd done it little by little throughout the year." Now's the time to adopt that approach, because the need for a CV, résumé, and portfolio doesn't end when your formal education ends. Once you're a practicing pharmacist, the challenge of keeping these items up to date only gets harder.

Keep the task manageable by working on it incrementally. Then you'll have everything you need when it's time for a performance review, career change, or something else that might require these materials.

I keep several versions of my CV on file in my computer at all times:

− A "final" version in both Word and PDF that may not have been updated for a few months but has been thoroughly checked for grammar, format, spelling, and punctuation. If I need to provide a copy quickly, the final version is always ready to go.
− A "draft update" that includes recent revisions. When I teach a class, give a presentation, or complete a publication that merits being added to my CV, I enter it quickly into the "draft update" version without worrying about formatting and grammar. Every few months I review and polish the "draft update" and it becomes my "final" version.

These two versions are chronologically complete, containing items all the way back to pharmacy school, including my experiential rotations. When I need a revised CV that contains selected information most relevant for the particular purpose, I go to the "final" version and remove unnecessary items. I then save the document with a title that reminds me of the purpose that version was used for. If I need a similar one later, it's already prepared and easy to find. Keeping a chronologically complete version on hand means I never have to worry that I removed items from my CV that I now want to put back.

I also keep several older versions of my CV, just in case, with the associated month and year listed. These have come in handy when I'm helping pharmacy students and residents prepare their own résumés and CVs, allowing me to pull up versions from a comparable time in my life. The list of files in my computer's CV folder looks roughly like this:
− CV draft update 04.10
− CV final 01.10
− CV 04.08
− CV 08.07
− CV 08.07 job interview at NHRMC
− CV 03.07

I use a similar approach to keeping my portfolio updated, but rather than using an electronic file, I use a physical one—a box. In the corner of my office is a cardboard box where I put copies of items that need to be added to my portfolio: PowerPoint presentations, certificates from completed programs, thank-you notes from patients and colleagues. Periodically I set aside time to organize and file the items in my portfolio binder.

To keep my presentations updated for both my portfolio and CV, I've gotten in the habit of making an extra copy of the handout while I'm making copies for attendees. As soon as I can, I add the name of the presentation to the "draft update" version of my CV and throw a copy of the handout into the box in my office. Later on, when I'm not in a hurry, I can add the handout to my portfolio and double check the formatting of my CV.

Interview Periodically

I perform a job search and try to interview for a new job approximately once a year, and I recommend that you do the same. Benefits include keeping your interviewing skills honed, staying on top of the types of jobs available, and remaining competitive for future career opportunities. Don't waste time by picking any pharmacy position that's available—that doesn't benefit you or the prospective employer. Employ the approaches described in chapters 3, 4, and 5. Be realistic and limit your search to areas of practice and geography you could truly see yourself going into.

For example, last year I specifically looked for a position similar to my current role that would allow me more patient interaction and direct patient care opportunities. I decided that I was unwilling to move outside of North Carolina, so I limited my search to administrative positions with a patient care component inside the state. Had no positions fitting that description been available, I would have browsed a bit more to see what kinds of jobs *were* posted. However, I found one position that seemed to fit the bill in another city where I have close family living. I decided to interview.

In my opinion, this type of job search and interview is much less stressful than the ones when you're exiting pharmacy school or residency. I was offered the new position, and all I had to do was compare it with my current job to determine which would meet my needs better. Both positions were *excellent* opportunities and the decision was difficult, but I chose to stay with my current position. So my interview didn't result in a change, but it boosted my confidence that my current position is best for me at this stage of my career.

Take the Time to Reflect

Periodically reflect on where you are in your career, your role as a pharmacist, and your trajectory for the future. Sometimes ethical dilemmas that you'll face as a health care professional will require you to reflect on how you feel about the situation and determine the right thing to do. These situations may be difficult and complicated. Remember to keep the thoughts and feelings of all involved parties in mind when making your decision, and put the best interests of the patient first. The textbook *Ethical Responsibility in Pharmacy Practice,* 2nd edition, is a great resource to help you reflect on ethical issues (Buerki RA, Vottero LD. Madison, Wis: American Institute of the History of Pharmacy; 2002).

Reflect on professionalism, too. In our day-to-day routines it's easy to forget all those things we promised when entering the profession, particularly if we don't care directly for patients. I'm not saying that over time, without conscious effort, we become more unprofessional; I'm saying that we must remember our role in the bigger picture. Several resources on professionalism are available at www.pharmacist.com in the Leadership and Professionalism Section of the APhA Academy of Student Pharmacists website.

One way I've found to review my obligations as a pharmacist is to incorporate a brief discussion of professionalism into the orientation for students whom I precept. I give a notebook to each student on rotation containing important documents, passwords, phone numbers, background readings, and other information, including the Oath of a Pharmacist (see Box 10-1) and the Code of Ethics for Pharmacists (see Box 10-2). As I walk through the binder with the students, I point out how easy it can be to temporarily lose sight of the bigger picture—and I remind them (and myself) to reflect.

Reflect on your long-term goals, as well. If you don't, you may wake up someday and realize you've let 10 or 20 years pass without actively reviewing where you're headed in your career—and whether it's where you'd intended to go. By virtue of completing a doctorate-level degree program, you've proven that you're highly motivated to perform well and be successful, but with no one measuring your performance the way they did in school—with no "next class" or "next exam"—you may lose some drive or focus.

When I was a resident, an important mentor suggested that I keep a list of goals in my PDA and review it regularly. My list included goals in these categories: professional, career, relationships (family and friends), travel, health and wellness, and financial. Some of these goals don't have a time limit, such as "take a multivitamin daily," while others include a suggested deadline.

Your list should always be a work in progress. Over time, as you review your goals, be flexible. Change the dates and reorganize items as your plans, priorities, and situation change.

Box 10-1

Oath of a Pharmacist

"I promise to devote myself to a lifetime of service to others through the profession of pharmacy. In fulfilling this vow:
- I will consider the welfare of humanity and relief of suffering my primary concerns.
- I will apply my knowledge, experience, and skills to the best of my ability to assure optimal outcomes for my patients.
- I will respect and protect all personal and health information entrusted to me.
- I will accept the lifelong obligation to improve my professional knowledge and competence.
- I will hold myself and my colleagues to the highest principles of our profession's moral, ethical, and legal conduct.
- I will embrace and advocate changes that improve patient care.
- I will utilize my knowledge, skills, experiences, and values to prepare the next generation of pharmacists.

I take these vows voluntarily with the full realization of the responsibility with which I am entrusted by the public."

Box 10-2

Code of Ethics for Pharmacists

A *pharmacist* respects the covenantal relationship between the patient and pharmacist.

A *pharmacist* promotes the good of every patient in a caring, compassionate, and confidential manner.

A *pharmacist* respects the autonomy and dignity of each patient.

A *pharmacist* acts with honesty and integrity in professional relationships.

A *pharmacist* maintains professional competence.

A *pharmacist* respects the values and abilities of colleagues and other health professionals.

A *pharmacist* serves individual, community, and societal needs.

A *pharmacist* seeks justice in the distribution of health resources.

Use Reverse Goal Setting

In her book *Devil with a Briefcase: 101 Success Secrets for the Spiritual Entrepreneur,* life coach Jan Janzen talks about "reverse goal setting," in which you envision the end result and work backwards to plan for a great outcome.

For example, if you want to become dean of a pharmacy school, think backwards. Start with the day you are appointed dean, and think, what has to happen the year before that? And then the year before that? Continue in this vein until you get to a goal you can start working on this year. Then identify a goal that you can start working on this month, then this week, then today. Write these goals down along the way. When you're done, you have written a roadmap for reaching your goal.

You can apply the same principle to most long term goals, whether for your career or your personal life. I use this approach when I advise residents on their residency project. I have them start with the end result—the presentation of their research— and write out what should happen just before that (practicing the presentation) and just before that (preparing the presentation) until all that's left is putting time frames on each step. Now the resident has a complete project plan and schedule.

Explore Additional Education and Credentials

Depending on your long-term career goals, additional education or credentials could be an opportunity for you to demonstrate an advanced skill set. These skills may set you apart from others, make you more competitive for your dream job, allow you to perform at a higher level of expertise, and otherwise enhance your role as a health care professional. Possible certifications include:
- Board of Pharmacy Specialties (BPS) (www.bpsweb.org)
  - Nuclear Pharmacy
  - Nutrition Support Pharmacy
  - Oncology Pharmacy
  - Pharmacotherapy
  - Psychiatric Pharmacy
- Certified Diabetes Educator (CDE) (www.ncbde.org)
- Board Certified in Advanced Diabetes Management (BC-ADM) (www.diabeteseducator.org)
- Certified Asthma Educator (AE-C) (www.naecb.org)

The certification most commonly pursued by pharmacists is Board-Certified Pharmacotherapy Specialist (BCPS), which is bestowed when you successfully complete the BPS pharmacotherapy exam. It's the most general of the certifications listed above and is intended for pharmacists who handle direct patient care, often function as part of a multidisciplinary team, and are often the main source of drug information for other health care professionals. The other certifications listed pertain to a specific disease state or area of specialty therapy.

Typically, these certifications require you to take an examination and meet a set of eligibility prerequisites. For example, to sit for the BCPS certification exam, the candidate must meet the following criteria:
— Graduation from a pharmacy program accredited by the Accreditation Council for Pharmacy Education (ACPE) or from a program outside the U.S. that qualifies the individual to practice in the jurisdiction.
— Current, active license to practice pharmacy in the U.S. or another jurisdiction.
— Completion of three years of practice experience with at least 50% of time spent in pharmacotherapy activities (as defined by the BPS Pharmacotherapy Content Outline) or completion of a PGY1 residency.

Maintaining these certifications can require a significant commitment, such as meeting CE or reexamination requirements, so make sure you carefully weigh the decision to pursue a credential. For example, the BCPS requires recertification every seven years, which consists of:
— Achieving a passing score on the 100-item, multiple-choice objective recertification examination, or...
— Earning 120 hours of CE credit provided by a professional development program approved by BPS.

If a credential will enhance your practice or help you achieve your professional goals, seriously consider pursuing it. The websites listed above provide specific information. Another great reference is the article, "Specialty Certifications Await After Graduation" (Keating J. *Student Pharmacist*. January/February 2004:24).

Stay Up to Date

After you leave school, it's a constant challenge to stay up to date with newly released literature and the rapidly changing world of health care. You can *actively* receive information by going out and finding it, or you can *passively* receive it through journals, newsletters, and other materials that come directly to you. Table 10-1 gives an overview of active and passive forms of information. For each type of information, decide how important it is and prioritize your time accordingly. For most incoming information, I follow the decision process illustrated in Figure 10-1.

Table 10-1

Active vs. Passive Collection of Information

Active	Passive
– Watching news on TV – Listening to news on the radio – Scanning your local newspaper in print or online – Scanning a national newspaper published daily in print or online – Scanning an international daily newspaper (such as *The New York Times*) in print or online – Checking health news websites, such as www.reutershealth.com – Using search engines, such as Medline or PubMed, to search primary literature – Using drug information resources, such as Micromedex – Continuing education programs	– Bulletins, newsletters, and/or emails from regulatory bodies and/or professional associations – *Pharmacist's Letter* – Professional journals you subscribe to or receive because of memberships in professional organizations – Email notifications from journals to which you do not subscribe that provide the table of contents for the most recent issue – Email newsletters from websites such as Medscape – Listserves – RSS feeds

Adapted from: http://itp.pharmacy.dal.ca/Scenarios/Keeping_Up-to-Date.php

Figure 10-1

Decision Process for Collecting Information

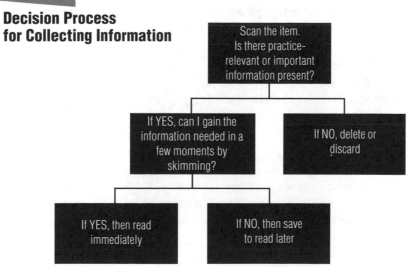

171

I keep a "save to read later" file folder in the bag I carry with me, so if a meeting starts late or I'm stuck somewhere waiting, I can pull out an item to read. Then I decide if the information is worth keeping.

There is no "one right way" to file information in your reference library, but you need some sort of consistent filing scheme, such as:
— An electronic file where you save materials that come in electronic format and place scanned copies of those that don't.
— A physical file of paper copies and printouts from electronic formats.

I use both. My preference is to keep electronic copies, but if an item doesn't come in that format, I keep a print copy.

Options for filing systems include:
— **A to Z File Cabinet.** Label file folders for each topic and arrange the folders alphabetically in the cabinet. This method is simple and easy, but may lead to some confusion in filing. For example, does an article on the use of beta-blockers in heart failure go in the "Beta-Blocker" file or the "Heart Failure" file?

— **A to Z Drugs and Disease States.** Alternatively, you could keep two files—one with folders for disease states and another with folders for drugs and drug classes. This can eliminate some of the confusion that comes with the A to Z method.

— **Alphanumeric Filing Scheme.** You can also use an alphanumeric filing scheme in which each major category has an abbreviation, minor categories have numbers, and subcategories add decimal places after the number. Here's an example from the website of the Dalhousie University School of Pharmacy, where you can find a more detailed explanation of the alphanumeric filing system (http://pharmacy.dal.ca/Resources/Filing_Scheme.php).

> QR = Quick Reference
> C = Community Pharmacy Topics
> H = Hospital/Institutional Pharmacy Topics

> Here's how numbers can be applied to the Quick Reference category:

> QR : QUICK REFERENCE (Section)
> QR60   Drug Interactions (Category)
> QR60.05   Drug-Drug Interactions (Subcategory)
> QR60.05.05 Drug Interactions with Oral Contraceptives (Sub-subcategory)

The more information you choose to keep, the more comprehensive your filing system should be. If you only have a few items to file, the A to Z system should be sufficient. If you keep a great deal of information, setting up an alphanumeric system should save you time locating information in your files.

Box 10-3 suggests further reading to help in your efforts to stay up to date.

Further Reading for Staying Up to Date

Health Care Informatics: A Skills-Based Resource
(Felkey BG, Fox BI, Thrower MR. Washington, D.C.: American Pharmacists Association; 2006.)
The practical information in this book helps health professionals and students use computer-related tools in health care, including the Internet, telecommunications, health care information systems, point-of-care technology, literature retrieval, evidence-based medicine, patient education, information security, and computer hardware and software. Each chapter includes activities to help develop and apply health care informatics skills.

Principles of Scientific Literature Evaluation: Critiquing Clinical Drug Trials
(Ascione FJ. Washington, D.C.: American Pharmaceutical Association; 2001.)
The author uses a structured instructional approach for evaluating clinical drug trials, based on 20 years of experience teaching the subject to student pharmacists. Each of nine chapters discusses portions of a published drug study.

Stay Connected

Networking, in essence, is systematically developing and maintaining personal and professional contacts for mutual career benefits—a critical task in the small world of pharmacy. It's important to cultivate positive relationships and avoid burning bridges, because you never know when you will need someone's assistance in the future.

Just by attending pharmacy school, you've already begun to network—with professors, advisors, teaching assistants, schoolmates, classmates, and others at your university. To further develop your personal network, consider these tips adapted from "Networking for Career Success" at www.pharmacist.com.

Become Active in Professional Associations

Get involved at the local, state, and/or national levels. Attend conferences, serve on committees, and volunteer your services. Offering to do the grunt work when serving on a committee will build favors and a positive reputation for yourself.

Be Organized

Carry a notebook or handheld computer to record the names, titles, addresses, and telephone numbers of contacts. Collect business cards and file them alphabetically according to areas of expertise. Write on the back of the card:

— Information that will help you remember where you met the person.
— How the person might be able to help you.
— Follow-up that you may have promised to undertake during your conversation.

I do both. I carry a handheld computer with my records, but rather than enter all contact information when I meet someone, I take their card, write pertinent information on it, as described above, and input the contact to my PDA at a later time. Be sure to carry business cards with you regularly, as well, so you're always prepared to quickly share your own information.

Follow Up with Contacts

Let people with whom you network know how leads they gave you turned out. No need to send a formal letter; handwritten notes or telephone calls are usually better because of their personal touch. Don't forget to make notations in your records of any written correspondence or calls. When anyone in your network of contacts achieves something professionally, write him or her a note of congratulations.

Use Good Manners

Always be polite and listen to what contacts have to say. Don't waste their time—be direct and specific when seeking help or information, and respect their busy schedules. Be sure to send a thank-you note to anyone who referred you to a job or professional opportunity. Many people forget this—remembering only to thank the interviewer and overlooking the person who helped them get the interview in the first place.

Nurture Your Networking Contacts

If you get in touch with people only when you need something, they'll quickly pick up on it and will no longer want to help you. Networking should work two ways. You support your contacts by giving them constructive feedback, providing information, introducing them to key people, and referring them to professional opportunities. In return, they will do the same for you.

Use Current Contacts to Find New Ones

When interacting with people, ask them to refer you to others in the field. As a young pharmacist, I often tagged along with mentors or fellow new practitioners and requested that they introduce me to key people, when appropriate. If you do this, use the name of the first person as a reference when contacting the second person.

Be Sincere

You have to be genuinely interested in, and conversant about, subjects that are dear to the contact. If you're not sincere, it will come across quickly and you'll lose that person's goodwill, leaving you worse off than if you had never approached him or her in the first place.

Volunteer

Get involved in a community volunteer clearinghouse or other volunteer organization and offer your time, skills, or advice to organizations, boards, and committees that need your help. You can also seek opportunities to volunteer or be a guest speaker for civic organizations and other groups. Volunteering is one of the best ways to get your name out there and make a good impression.

I found the pharmacy at my local free clinic to be a great place to volunteer and network. Now I not only volunteer there, I've also established a collaborative practice and I serve on the organization's board of directors, bringing me even more networking opportunities.

Joining my local emergency response team was also an excellent way for me to meet new people from other professions. Our team is called upon to respond to local, state, and national disasters (such as Hurricane Katrina) to set up mobile field hospitals and care for patients. As a member of this team, called an SMAT II team, I train one Saturday every other month alongside volunteer pharmacists and other professionals to prepare for possible deployments. As a result, I have a great local network of pharmacists, nurses, physicians, emergency medical technicians, and firefighters.

Maintain and Build School Contacts

Keep in touch with former teachers and professors. Ask them to let you know who the up-and-coming professionals are or to alert you to opportunities in your field.

Contact your school's career center or alumni association. Find out if they sponsor networking and social opportunities and get on the mailing list. I found that serving on my school's alumni association board of directors was a great way to get involved after graduation.

Contact Published Professionals

When reading professional publications, keep a close eye on the names of authors and people mentioned who share your interests or goals, and think about how you could get to know them. You could pave the way by sending them a note about an issue of mutual concern. This approach may seem intimidating—you may worry about bothering the person—but I've never had a poor result from this type of interaction. Most often, authors are flattered that you've read their publication and will be happy to discuss it with you in further detail or answer your questions about their work.

Find and Be a Mentor

You need many mentors, commonly defined as trusted counselors or guides. You can benefit from a wide range of relationships throughout your career with people who are more experienced than you. Undoubtedly you'll meet people you admire for many different reasons. You might turn to one mentor for advice on professional development; to another for clinical mentorship in your area of practice; and to yet another for advice in maintaining work–life balance.

As with your networking contacts, you must respect your mentors' time and use good manners, be sincere, and so on. There isn't just one correct way to pursue a mentoring relationship. Sometimes people in that role aren't fully aware of it and never use the term "mentor" with you. Others may fill a more formal mentoring role in your life. Some you may talk to periodically; others you may see regularly.

Mentors can be fellow pharmacists, other health care professionals, neighbors, acquaintances, or other people you meet along your professional journey. Although the following suggestions might not apply to all mentoring situations, they provide some structure for a rewarding and useful relationship.
- Try to set a regular time for meetings (by phone or in person).
- Take control of maintaining regular contact.
- Prepare for your meetings beforehand so you don't waste valuable time.
- Don't make too many demands on your mentor's time. They are busy people who are giving up their time to help you. If you need to cancel a meeting, give them notice, and be reasonable about contacting them during their workday or personal time.
- Learn from the guidance your mentor gives you. Be open to suggestions and try out their ideas. Tell your mentor if you acted on his or her advice and explain the outcome.
- Provide feedback and do what you say you are going to do. Your mentor needs to know that you are interested in developing your skills and making use of his or her knowledge, which will help maintain a strong relationship.

– Give something back to your mentor whenever you can, such as sharing valuable information or providing useful contacts.

You should also seek to be a mentor, even if you don't see yourself as an exceptionally skilled or seasoned health care professional. There is always someone less skilled than you who could use your guidance. You've certainly been through experiences and learned things that can benefit others. You can even be a mentor in one area of a person's life (such as helping her train for a marathon) while she serves as a mentor for you in another (helping you improve your patient counseling skills).

A great way to launch your role as a mentor is to precept students. Let them know they can always contact you after their rotations are complete if they have questions or need advice. You can also volunteer with your local health profession's educators and community organizations to provide information and advice to others. I've built relationships with mentees by letting them shadow me at work or volunteer in my practice. I've also gone to local high schools to lead discussions about careers in pharmacy. Box 10-4 lists further resources on mentoring. You'll find that being both a mentee and a mentor will greatly enhance your life.

Box 10-4

Further Resources on Mentoring

How to Find and Succeed as a Mentor
(White SJ, Tryon JE. *Am J Health Syst Pharm*. Jun 2007; 64:1258-9.)
In this article, the authors discuss successful ways to find a mentor and be an effective mentor.

Making the Most of Being Mentored: How to Grow from a Mentoring Partnership
(Shea GF. Menlo Park, Calif: Crisp; 1999.)
This book teaches how to create and grow from a mentor/mentee partnership and includes techniques for maximizing results.

The Mentee's Guide to Mentoring
(Cohen NH. Amherst, Mass: Human Resource Development Press; 1999.)
The art of establishing and maintaining productive interpersonal communication with mentors is covered, so mentees can contribute as much as possible. Each of 15 sections contains concise information about an important aspect of the mentoring experience.

continued on page 178

Box 10-4

continued

Mentoring Exchange
(www.ashp.org)
This service for members of the American Society of Health-System Pharmacists
(ASHP) lets you sign up online to be a mentor or a mentee. Each fills out a profile; then
mentees can browse and request specific mentors, who have the option of accepting or
declining. The site also contains helpful information about mentoring.

Mentoring Information Kit
(www.educause.edu/mentoring)
This online kit is from EDUCAUSE, a nonprofit association that advances higher education
by promoting the intelligent use of information technology. The site has information about
mentoring in general as well as specific sections geared toward mentees and mentors.

Power Mentoring: How Successful Mentors and Protégés Get the Most Out of Their Relationships
(Ensher EA, Murphy SE. San Francisco: Jossey-Bass; 2005.)
This nuts-and-bolts guide for anyone who wants to connect with a protégé or mentor
or improve a mentoring relationship includes examples and insights from 50 of
America's most successful mentors and protégés.

Tips for Mentees and Mentors from the Mentoring Group
(www.mentoringgroup.com/html/archive.html)
A division of the not-for-profit Coalition of Counseling Centers, Inc., the Mentoring
Group has a website that offers dozens of articles on the essentials of mentoring, best
practices, how to mentor over a distance, and being an effective mentee.

What's Next After You Say Hello: First Steps in Mentoring
(Hogue WF, Pringle EM. *EDUCAUSE Quarterly.* 2005;28[2]:50–52.)
This article covers creating a co-mentoring relationship with mutuality and clear goals,
so everyone involved benefits.

Pharmacy Organizations

Many different associations have been established over the years to serve the interests of pharmacists, promote pharmacists' education and growth, and support the pharmacy profession. Key national and international pharmacy associations are listed here in alphabetical order; in addition, each state has its own pharmacy association to serve as a resource to pharmacists licensed and practicing within that state.

Academy of Managed Care Pharmacy (AMCP)
www.amcp.org
AMCP is geared toward pharmacists and other health care practitioners who serve people covered by managed care pharmacy benefits.

American Association of Colleges of Pharmacy (AACP)
www.aacp.org
AACP represents pharmacy education and educators in the United States.

American College of Clinical Pharmacy (ACCP)
www.accp.com
ACCP is a professional and scientific society that provides leadership, education, advocacy, and resources for clinical pharmacists.

American College of Veterinary Pharmacists (ACVP)
www.vetmeds.org
ACVP supports independent pharmacists who provide services to veterinarians.

American Pharmacists Association (APhA)
www.pharmacist.com
APhA, the earliest established national professional society of pharmacists in the United States, represents pharmacists from all practice settings and scientific disciplines.

American Society of Consultant Pharmacists (ASCP)
www.ascp.com
ASCP represents pharmacists who have expertise in providing medication therapy management and distribution services to seniors in long-term care facilities, assisted living facilities, and home care.

American Society of Health-System Pharmacists (ASHP)
www.ashp.org
ASHP represents pharmacists who practice in hospitals, health maintenance organizations, long-term care facilities, home care, and other components of health care systems.

Association of Natural Medicine Pharmacists (ANMP)
www.anmp.org
ANMP serves pharmacists and others interested in the field of natural medicine.

College of Psychiatric and Neurologic Pharmacists (CPNP)
www.cpnp.org
CPNP's mission is to optimize treatment outcomes of people affected by psychiatric and neurologic disorders.

International Pharmaceutical Federation (FIP)
www.fip.org
FIP is an international federation of national associations representing pharmaceutical practitioners and scientists.

National Community Pharmacists Association (NCPA)
www.ncpanet.org
NCPA represents independent community pharmacy in the United States.

Society of Infectious Diseases Pharmacists (SIDP)
www.sidp.org
SIDP is an association of pharmacists and other health care professionals dedicated to promoting the appropriate use of antimicrobials.

INDEX

Note: Italicized letters *b*, *f*, and *t* following page numbers indicate boxes, figures, and tables, respectively.

		DATE DUE	